Evidence-Based School Psychiatry

Guest Editors

JEFFREY Q. BOSTIC, MD, EdD
ALEXA L. BAGNELL, MD, FRCPC

CHILD AND ADOLESCENT PSYCHIATRIC CLINICS OF NORTH AMERICA

www.childpsych.theclinics.com

Consulting Editor
HARSH K. TRIVEDI, MD

January 2012 • Volume 21 • Number 1

SAUNDERS an imprint of ELSEVIER, Inc.

W.B. SAUNDERS COMPANY
A Division of Elsevier Inc.

Elsevier Inc. • 1600 John F. Kennedy Boulevard • Suite 1800 • Philadelphia, Pennsylvania 19103-2899

http://www.childpsych.theclinics.com

CHILD AND ADOLESCENT PSYCHIATRIC CLINICS OF NORTH AMERICA Volume 21, Number 1
January 2012 ISSN 1056–4993, ISBN-13: 978-1-4557-3839-7

Editor: Sarah E. Barth

Child and Adolescent Psychiatric Clinics of North America (ISSN 1056-4993) is published quarterly by Elsevier Inc., 360 Park Avenue South, New York, NY 10010-1710. Months of issue are January, April, July, and October. Business and Editorial Offices: 1600 John F. Kennedy Boulevard, Suite 1800, Philadelphia, PA 19103-2899. Periodicals postage paid at New York, NY and additional mailing offices. Subscription prices are $297.00 per year (US individuals), $453.00 per year (US institutions), $150.00 per year (US students), $343.00 per year (Canadian individuals), $546.00 per year (Canadian institutions), $190.00 per year (Canadian students), $408.00 per year (international individuals), $546.00 per year (international institutions), and $190.00 per year (international students). International air speed delivery is included in all *Clinics* subscription prices. All prices are subject to change without notice. **POSTMASTER:** Send address changes to *Child and Adolescent Psychiatric Clinics of North America,* Elsevier Health Sciences Division, Subscription Customer Service, 3251 Riverport Lane, Maryland Heights, MO 63043. **Customer Service: 1-800-654-2452 (U.S. and Canada); 314-447-8871 (outside U.S. and Canada). Fax: 314-447-8029. E-mail: JournalsCustomerService-usa@ elsevier.com (for print support) or journalsonlinesupport-usa@elsevier.com (for online support).**

Reprints. For copies of 100 or more of articles in this publication, please contact the Commercial Reprints Department, Elsevier Inc., 360 Park Avenue South, New York, New York 10010-1710 Tel.: (212) 633-3812; Fax: (212) 462-1935, e-mail: reprints@elsevier.com.

Child and Adolescent Psychiatric Clinics of North America is covered in *MEDLINE/PubMed (Index Medicus), ISI, SSCI, Research Alert, Social Search, Current Contents,* and *EMBASE/Excerpta Medica.*

Printed and bound by CPI Group (UK) Ltd, Croydon, CR0 4YY
Transferred to Digital Print 2012

Contributors

CONSULTING EDITOR

HARSH K. TRIVEDI, MD
Associate Professor of Psychiatry, Vanderbilt University School of Medicine; and Executive Medical Director, and Chief of Staff, Vanderbilt Psychiatric Hospital, Nashville, Tennessee

CONSULTING EDITOR EMERITUS

ANDRÉS MARTIN, MD, MPH

FOUNDING CONSULTING EDITOR

MELVIN LEWIS, MBBS, FRCPSYCH, DCH

GUEST EDITORS

JEFFREY Q. BOSTIC, MD, EdD
Associate Clinical Professor, Department of Psychiatry, Harvard Medical School; Director of School Psychiatry, Massachusetts General Hospital, Boston, Massachusetts

ALEXA L. BAGNELL, MD, FRCPC
Associate Professor, Department of Psychiatry, Dalhousie University, Halifax, Nova, Scotia; IWK Maritime Psychiatry, Nova Scotia, Canada

AUTHORS

ALEXA L. BAGNELL, MD, FRCPC
Associate Professor, Department of Psychiatry, Dalhousie University, Halifax, Nova, Scotia; IWK Maritime Psychiatry, Nova Scotia, Canada

SHILPA BAWEJA, MS
Graduate Student Researcher, Department of Psychiatry and Biobehavioral Sciences, University of California, Los Angeles, Semel Institute, Health Services Research Center, Los Angeles, California

JEFFREY Q. BOSTIC, MD, EdD
Associate Clinical Professor, Department of Psychiatry, Harvard Medical School; Director of School Psychiatry, Massachusetts General Hospital, Boston, Massachusetts

COLBY BRUNT, JD
Partner, Stoneman, Chandler, & Miller LLP

ALISON L. CALEAR, PhD
Centre for Mental Health Research, The Australian National University, Acton, Australian Capital Territory, Australia

RICARDO B. EIRALDI, PhD
Assistant Professor, Department of Pediatrics, University of Pennsylvania, Perelman School of Medicine; Department of Child and Adolescent Psychiatry and Behavioral Sciences, The Children's Hospital of Philadelphia, Philadelphia, Pennsylvania

ELIZABETH K. ENGLANDER, PhD
Director, Massachusetts Aggression Reduction Center, Bridgewater State University, Bridgewater, Massachusetts

LAUREN J. HART, BS
Department of Psychiatry, Harvard Medical School; Department of Public Health, Northeastern University, Boston, Massachusetts

MIKE S. JELLINEK, MD
Chief, Child Psychiatry, Massachusetts General Hospital; Professor of Psychiatry and of Pediatrics, Harvard Medical School, Boston; President, Newton Wellesley Hospital, Newton, Massachusetts

SHERYL KATAOKA, MD, MSHS
Associate Professor, Department of Psychiatry and Biobehavioral Sciences, Center for Health Services and Society, Semel Institute, University of California, Los Angeles, California

STAN KUTCHER, MD, FRCPC, FCAHS
Sun Life Financial Chair in Adolescent Mental Health; Director, WHO/PAHO Collaborating Centre in Mental Health Training and Policy Development; Professor of Psychiatry, Dalhousie University and the IWK Health Centre, Halifax, Nova Scotia, Canada

AUDRA K. LANGLEY, PhD
Assistant Professor, Department of Psychiatry and Biobehavioral Sciences, Center for Health Services and Society, Semel Institute, University of California, Los Angeles, California

TERRY LEE, MD
Assistant Professor, Public Behavioral Health and Justice Policy Division, Department of Psychiatry and Behavioral Sciences, University of Washington School of Medicine, Seattle, Washington

KATHARINA MANASSIS, MD, FRCPC
Professor of Psychiatry, University of Toronto, Department of Psychiatry, Hospital for Sick Children, Toronto, Ontario, Canada

JENNIFER A. MAUTONE, PhD
Clinical and Research Psychologist, Department of Child and Adolescent Psychiatry and Behavioral Sciences, The Children's Hospital of Philadelphia, Philadelphia, Pennsylvania

UCHENWA D. OKOLI, MD
Senior Resident, Child Psychiatry Service, Massachusetts General Hospital; Clinical Fellow, Harvard Medical School, Boston, Massachusetts

THOMAS J. POWER, PhD
Professor, Department of Pediatrics, University of Pennsylvania, Perelman School of Medicine; Department of Child and Adolescent Psychiatry and Behavioral Sciences, The Children's Hospital of Philadelphia, Philadelphia, Pennsylvania

JEFFERSON B. PRINCE, MD
Director of Child Psychiatry, MassGeneral for Children at North Shore Medical Center, Salem; Staff Pediatric Psychopharmacology Clinic, Massachusetts General Hospital; Instructor in Psychiatry, Harvard Medical School, Boston, Massachusetts

JULIE L. RYAN, PhD
Assistant Professor, School of Psychology, Fairleigh Dickinson University, Teaneck, New Jersey

DARCY A. SANTOR, PhD
Professor, School of Psychology, University of Ottawa, Ottawa, Ontario, Canada

BRADLEY D. STEIN, MD, PhD
Health Services Researcher, RAND Corporation; Associate Professor of Psychiatry, University of Pittsburgh School of Medicine, Pittsburgh, Pennsylvania

JONATHAN R. STEVENS, MD, MPH
Medical Director, Pediatric Inpatient Psychiatry Unit, MassGeneral for Children at North Shore Medical Center, Salem, Massachusetts

CARRIE MASIA WARNER, PhD
Associate Professor of Child and Adolescent Psychiatry and Pediatrics, NYU Langone Medical Center, New York, New York; Associate Director of the Anita Saltz Institute for Anxiety and Mood Disorders, NYU Child Study Center, New York; Research Scientist, Nathan Kline Institute for Psychiatric Research, Orangeburg, New York

YIFENG WEI, Med, PhD Candidate
Sun Life Financial Chair in Adolescent Mental Health, Dalhousie University and IWK Health Centre, Halifax, Nova Scotia, Canada

MARLEEN WONG, PhD
Assistant Dean and Clinical Professor of Field Education, University of Southern California, School of Social Work, Los Angeles, California

AMY M. YULE, MD
Department of Psychiatry, Massachusetts General Hospital, Boston, Massachusetts

Contents

Contemporary Topics and Current State of Knowledge

Youth mental health is increasingly recognized as a key concern with significant impact on youth and society. School is the one setting where professionals are consistently available to monitor how children are functioning and learning and intervene and support. School psychiatry has expanded beyond individual mental health problems to school-wide and community issues including school violence, sexual harassment, bullying, substance abuse, discrimination, and discipline. This article describes the importance of mental health literacy in health outcomes and research in school-based mental health programs to better position the clinician to advocate at the individual and/or system level.

School mental health programs from developed countries demonstrate that both the practice and research are becoming more important to policy makers, educators, health providers, parents, and other stakeholders. Some United Nations agencies and other international organizations have begun work to advance school mental health internationally. School-based mental health programming needs to be considered as part of usual child and youth mental health policies and plans, whether those are national or other jurisdictional in nature. Currently, a paucity of evidence-based and cost effective child and youth global mental health policies/programs exist, limiting school-based mental health programs being developed, implemented, or sustained.

Schools are evolving to support all students, including those with mental health issues. Clinicians can help patients and schools by providing diagnostic clarity about a child's condition, how that condition interferes with school progress, and what interventions are needed in the school setting. State and Federal legislation supports timely response by schools to mental health issues emerging in students through special education laws and general education accommodations, such as Response To Intervention (RTI), which encourages schools to implement evidence-based interventions for students exhibiting mental health conditions. Case examples illuminate important legal considerations when clinicians are faced with issues such as therapeutic placements, home hospital forms, and substance abuse, and student misconduct.

schooling might be shaped with regard to children's and adolescents' brain development needs rather than social custom.

Clear benefits of school-based interventions focusing on health and mental health promotion or illness have been documented. A number of permanent repositories that rate and list effective school-based programs have been established. However, efforts to implement programs on a mass scale have not succeeded. There is a need to balance program development and improvement with uptake and implementation. This article outlines what is known about knowledge exchange and mobilization and introduces a business lens for school-based mental health programs uptake and sustainability. Individual clinicians can have significant impact by promoting strategies for both patients and the whole school population.

Evidence-Based School Approaches to Psychopathology

Interventions for students with generalized anxiety disorder require attention to contextual factors both within and outside the classroom. They often are based on the principles of increasing environmental predictability and increasing the student's sense of self-efficacy. Good judgment is sometimes needed to determine which strategies constitute reasonable accommodations to the student's anxiety and which constitute an excessive deviation from usual school expectations. The latter can single out students unnecessarily or limit their academic progress. Working closely with parents and mental health professionals involved in the student's care is most likely to ensure a consistently helpful approach.

As is evident from the topic of this issue, schools can play an important role in addressing the unmet mental health needs of youth. Social anxiety disorder is particularly suited to being treated in the school setting. This article describes an empirically supported school-based intervention for social anxiety disorder, skills for academic and social success, and provides specific strategies to school counselors, teachers and community practitioners for implementing these methods. This article focuses on practical approaches for working with socially anxious adolescents in the school setting and how to increase awareness of social anxiety with parents and school personnel.

> The prevalence of trauma exposure among youth is a major public health concern. Students who have experienced a traumatic event are at increased risk for academic, social, and emotional problems. School can be an ideal setting for mental health professionals to intervene with traumatized students, school staff, and parents both immediately following a traumatic event and when symptoms of posttraumatic stress disorder and other trauma-related mental health problems develop. This article describes evidence-based treatments for posttraumatic stress disorder and outlines practical approaches to use in schools.

> Depression is a prevalent and debilitating disorder that can severely affect a young person's social, emotional, and academic functioning. Identifying depression early is essential to reducing the impact of this disorder. Depression is treatable. However, there are a number of classroom and school supports that can be put in place to assist a young person experiencing or recovering from depression. Preventing the development of depression through effective classroom programs should be encouraged and supported within the school environment.

> An extensive amount of research has demonstrated the effectiveness of psychosocial interventions for children with ADHD. Historically, the research has focused on interventions targeting problems in the home or school setting, but more recent research has highlighted the importance of family – school partnerships and conjoint approaches to intervention involving family and school. Effective approaches to psychosocial intervention consist of strategies to address performance deficits, promote adaptive behavior, and improve children's self-control and academic and social skills. Considerable evidence exists to indicate that combined approaches are more effective in reducing ADHD symptoms and related academic and social impairments than separate treatments.

> Youth disruptive behavior is a concern for youth, school personnel, families, and society. Early childhood disruptive behaviors negatively

impact the classroom, and are associated with negative academic, social, behavioral, emotional, substance use, health, and justice system outcomes in adolescence and adulthood. Effective, comprehensive, multicomponent interventions targeting risk/protective factors and pathways associated with antisocial behavior reduce and/or mitigate these negative outcomes. Positive effects have been demonstrated for universal and indicated programs for participating youth and families in early childhood, and for high-risk youth in adolescence and young adulthood. These empirically supported programs inform the treatment of complex and difficult-to-treat disruptive behavior.

Adolescent substance use is a major public health problem that concerns parents, schools, clinicians, and policy makers. The authors review school-based prevention programs, school drug policies, clinical signs and symptoms of substance impairment, recommendations for referral and engaging adolescents who are using substances, and treatment interventions for adolescent substance use disorders.

The term **psychosis** is generally used to describe the abnormal behaviors of children and adolescents with grossly impaired reality testing. This article discusses evaluation of psychotic symptoms in students and psychosocial school interventions for students with psychosis, including the roles of teachers and school administrators. Psychoeducation provided by clinicians and school staff to enhance coping and cognitive strategies is described.

FORTHCOMING ISSUES

April 2012

Depression
Stuart J. Goldman, MD, and
Frances J. Wren, MB, MRC,
Guest Editors

July 2012

Anxiety Disorders
Moira A. Rynn, MD, Hilary Vidair, PhD,
and Jennifer U. Blackford, PhD,
Guest Editors

October 2012

Psychopharmacology
Harsh K. Trivedi, MD, and
Kiki Chang, MD, *Guest Editors*

RECENT ISSUES

October 2011

Gender Variant Childern and Transgender Adolescents
Richard R. Pleak, MD, *Guest Editor*

July 2011

Forensic Psychiatry
William Bernet, MD, and
Bradley W. Freeman, MD, *Guest Editors*

April 2011

Cognitive-Behavioral Therapy in Youth
Todd E. Peters, MD, and
Jennifer B. Freeman, PhD, *Guest Editors*

THE CLINICS ARE NOW AVAILABLE ONLINE!

Access your subscription at:
www.theclinics.com

Preface

Evidence-Based School Psychiatry

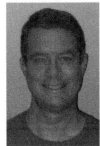
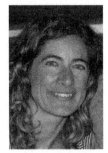

Jeffrey Q. Bostic, MD, EdD   Alexa L. Bagnell, MD, FRCPC
Guest Editors

Our patients engage with teachers, school counselors, and school administrators for approximately 15,000 hours during their childhood and adolescence. Partnering with these committed adults, instrumental in so many children's lives, only makes good sense. School success is a key factor in child and youth long-term outcomes and mental illness can significantly impact school functioning. While our patients sometimes have complicated constellations of symptoms that interfere with every aspect of their lives, schools afford a consistent and supportive setting for intervention unavailable anywhere else. While this process can be complicated, and some schools have more resource constraints than others, in most cases a teacher, coach, assistant principal, school nurse, or counselor within the building is positioned to help that child in a meaningful and effective way. School personnel are in an ideal position to recognize and intervene for children and youth with mental health difficulties and can be essential allies in changing the trajectory of the vulnerable population we serve.

Child psychiatry continues to flourish, to develop, to become more sophisticated in every arena, as psychopharmacology to psychotherapy techniques become more developmentally sensitive and disorder specific. School mental health has been identified as an emerging priority area globally by governments, researchers, clinicians, and educators. This volume provides a distillation of the current evidence-base in school psychiatry, prioritizing what information most matters to those working in the trenches. The authors are an international group of experts "doing" this work in schools. The articles are designed to be practical tools for clinicians, moving away from various programs or models (including their own) and instead toward "what classroom interventions most make a difference" for addressing anxiety, depression,

Child Adolesc Psychiatric Clin N Am 21 (2012) xiii–xvi
doi:10.1016/j.chc.2011.10.001
1056-4993/12/$ – see front matter © 2012 Elsevier Inc. All rights reserved.

inattention, mood regulation, vulnerability to substance abuse, bullying, etc. We have tried to find the best evidence-based support for addressing mental health symptoms in the classroom. Child psychiatrists can then use this information to advance knowledge and capacity in school personnel working with our patients to improve outcomes. While pharmacotherapy is a significant component of treatment for many of our patients, this volume does not focus on such treatments. Rather, this volume attempts to provide what is known in 2011 in terms of school-based interventions for mental health and mental illness that can be implemented by school personnel. Accordingly, while this volume was constructed with child psychiatrists as the primary audience, this volume will also be useful to school staff (including administrators), government (policymakers), and psychologists, social workers, and other clinicians who work with schools.

School psychiatry is a relatively new area of research with some strong evidence-based practices, particularly in addressing specific disorders (section 2), and with some emerging areas that clearly impact mental health outcomes in schools (section 1). Section 1, Contemporary Topics and Current State of Knowledge, includes topics on the frontier of our knowledge base that have broad population impact with direct relevance to mental health outcomes in children and youth. Section 2, Evidence-Based School Approaches to Psychopathology, provides disorder-specific recommendations from evidence-based research to support students with mental illness in the school setting.

Section 1 begins with the Bagnell and colleagues article on mental health literacy, shifting our paradigm to viewing mental health as requiring basic mental health literacy, with the factors important for basic mental health literacy as primary in our considerations as we work with schools, even one patient (student) at a time. Wei and Kutcher then describe the global state of school mental health, including recommendations to connect mental health with wider governmental and educational health agendas. Educational attorney Brunt then summarizes contemporary legal aspects for students with mental health issues, distinguishing between relevant Federal statutes and describing the "Response to Intervention" mandates that direct schools to implement research-based interventions promptly for students manifesting mental health conditions. Englander describes bullying and cyberbullying, how school practices may contribute to bullying, and recommended school responses to bullying types of behaviors. Jellinek describes how schools can mobilize and proceed when students die, amidst diverse circumstances. Bostic and Hart describe biological/psychological/social practices that schools may enact to promote mental health, including adjusting the school day schedule, practices found most (and least) effective for student achievement, and promoting mental health by focusing on variables associated with happiness. The last article in this section by Santor describes the variables important for sustaining meaningful changes within school as mental health interventions or programs are put in place.

Section 2 of this volume, Evidence-Based School Approaches to Psychopathology, addresses the mental health conditions that have been most studied in school settings, often with programs specific to anxiety, trauma, depression, etc, now in place. Each author describes important components for schools considering programs to address mental health issues and the evidence supporting these interventions. In addition, each author provides specific recommendations to help support and improve outcomes for students with these mental health conditions so that clinicians can provide evidence-based strategies to school staff regarding their patients.

The first three articles in this section address students with anxiety. Manassis describes cognitive-behavioral therapy-based school programs implemented to address generalized anxiety symptoms, and specific interventions to address topics such as perfectionism, fear of assignments, and test anxiety. Ryan and Masia-Warner describe effective components of two well-evaluated social anxiety school-based programs, and tactics for developing realistic thinking about social situations, facing social fears, and methods for exposures and reinforcement of desirable social skills to diminish social anxiety. Kataoka and colleagues describe five school-based programs to address posttraumatic stress disorder symptoms, and relevant psychoeducation supports, as well as specific techniques for those working with children exposed to trauma.

The remaining four articles address, respectively, student depression, attention-deficit hyperactivity disorder (ADHD), oppositional/conduct symptoms, substance abuse, and psychosis in the school setting. Calear examines the evidence base for depression prevention programs in school settings and describes specific program components including specific school modifications for students with depression. Eiraldi, Maurone, and Power describe interventions for students with ADHD, including schoolwide strategies such as Positive Behavioral Support, and individual strategies in the classroom for students with ADHD including reinforcement techniques and improving self-management strategies. Eiraldi and colleagues further address developmental differences to consider in recommendations and programming for students with ADHD. Lee describes the complex circumstances contributing to disruptive behavior conditions in students and describes the research base in comprehensive programs such as PATH/Fast Track, Seattle Social Development/Raising Healthy Children, and The Incredible Years. Lee details how behavior analysis can be used to address various disruptive or oppositional behaviors for individual students (eg, aggression at school, calling out in the classroom, refusing to do homework). Yule and Prince describe several prominent substance abuse prevention programs in schools, and the "key variables" of interventions that seem most important for diminishing student substance abuse. They review symptoms of substance abuse in schools, and pragmatic approaches for responding to and supporting students with substance use problems. Stevens addresses psychosis emerging in students and the important distinction between various conditions manifesting as psychosis, providing suggestions for clinicians to help schools plan around the wider needs of individual students exhibiting psychotic symptoms. School-based strategies to decrease and help students to cope better and manage psychotic symptoms are discussed.

Schools educate students and are increasingly recognized as fundamental in the social and emotional development of youth. To cultivate "mentally healthy" adults, schools are being asked to expand beyond the educational curriculum and provide an environment that supports mental health and wellness. These articles provide the current state of knowledge about enhancing mental health, inhibiting the evolution of mental health symptoms, and expanding the strategies and supports for students to manage anxiety, depression, inattention, trauma, substance use, and psychosis better. Admittedly, we are still on the frontier of our understanding of what best to advocate for in schools. However, there is clear evidence that improving the mental health of youth in schools is a necessary and fundamental factor in functional outcomes, and that psychiatrists are in a prime position to advocate for these changes and supports. There is enough science to start now, to partner up, and to ensure our recommendations for schools are empirically informed. Helping our youth succeed is a cooperative effort, and this volume provides clinicians the empirical tools to be an informed advocate and collaborator in this partnership.

Jeffrey Q. Bostic, MD, EdD
School Psychiatry
Massachusetts General Hospital
55 Fruit Street
Boston, MA 02114, USA

Alexa L. Bagnell, MD, FRCPC
Department of Psychiatry
Dalhousie University
IWK Maritime Psychiatry
5850/5980 University Avenue
Halifax, NS B3K 6R8, Canada

E-mail addresses:
JBOSTIC@PARTNERS.ORG (J.Q. Bostic)
Alexa.Bagnell@iwk.nshealth.ca (A.L. Bagnell)

Erratum

The publisher acknowledges an error in Dr Paul Bensussan's article, "Forensic Psychiatry in France: The Outreau Case and False Allegations of Child Sexual Abuse," which appeared in the July 2011 issue of *Child and Adolescent Psychiatric Clinics of North America,* Vol. 20, Number 3.

On page 522 of this article, the beginning of the last paragraph, the term *Cour de cassation* was used instead of *Cour d'assises*. *Cour de cassation* refers to the Supreme Court, whereas *Cour d'assises* is the Criminal Court. The sentence should read as follows:

"The convictions in the Outreau case were appealed to the *Cour d'assises* (Criminal Court) and the trial opened in Paris in November 2005."

Child Adolesc Psychiatric Clin N Am 21 (2012) xvii
doi:10.1016/j.chc.2011.10.002
1056-4993/12/$ – see front matter © 2012 Elsevier Inc. All rights reserved.

childpsych.theclinics.com

Building Mental Health Literacy: Opportunities and Resources for Clinicians

Alexa L. Bagnell, MD, FRCPC[a,*], Darcy A. Santor, PhD[b]

KEYWORDS

• School • Youth • Mental health literacy • Decision-making

Youth mental health is increasingly recognized as a key national health concern with significant impact on future outcomes for youth and society. There is growing awareness of the high prevalence of youth mental health problems, low rates of treatment, and high costs to youth and society of untreated mental illness in young people. In the school setting, youth with mental illness are more likely to have significant academic difficulties including disciplinary issues, absenteeism, failure, and school dropout.[1] Because most American youth attend school, school psychiatry has become an important arena for addressing the growing mental health needs of children and adolescents. Youth spend close to half of their waking hours each day in school. For most children, school is the one natural setting where professionals are consistently available to monitor how they are functioning and learning, and to intervene and support in almost aspects of their lives when necessary.

Teachers are trained to be educators and rarely have expertise in mental health. Yet because of the increasing prevalence of mental health disorders impacting school success in our youth and legislation mandating schools meet these needs, there is growing demand for both mental health education and prevention/intervention strategies for youth within schools. Recognition of problem behaviors among students such as substance abuse, unprotected sexual intercourse, and, more recently, bullying and school violence has led schools to turn to mental health clinicians for clarity and direction. Research in the area of school psychiatry in the past two decades has been increasing with programs targeting specific mental health disorders as well as broader emotional and behavioral whole-school program approaches.

The role of the psychiatrist has also evolved over time to recognize the importance of schools in mental health treatment and prevention outcomes. Psychiatrists demonstrate a wide range of mental health involvement in the school setting. This

[a] Department of Psychiatry, Dalhousie University, Halifax, Nova Scotia, Canada
[b] School of Psychology, University of Ottawa, Ottawa, ON, Canada
* Corresponding author. Izaak Walton Killam (IWK) Health Centre, Maritime Psychiatry, 5850/5980 University Avenue, Halifax, NS, B3K 6R8, Canada.
E-mail address: Alexa.Bagnell@iwk.nshealth.ca

Child Adolesc Psychiatric Clin N Am 21 (2012) 1–9
doi:10.1016/j.chc.2011.09.007
1056-4993/12/$ – see front matter © 2012 Elsevier Inc. All rights reserved.

childpsych.theclinics.com

involvement can range from individual consultation with a student-patient and developing a plan to meet patient needs, which may include school interventions, to systemic approaches including early intervention and prevention programming within a school district more generally.

School psychiatry has expanded beyond individual mental health problems to address school-wide and community issues including school violence, sexual harassment, bullying, substance abuse, discrimination, and discipline. This introduction provides an overview of the importance of mental health literacy in health outcomes and the research in school-based mental health programs to better position the clinician to advocate at the individual and/or system level.

THE CHALLENGE

Schools today face great demands to inculcate knowledge, to prepare students with vocational skills, to socialize children to interact with others appropriately, and to meet their health, emotional, and behavioral needs that impact their learning. The health crisis in youth (eg, obesity, mental illness, substance misuse/abuse) seems greater than ever before. The demands far exceed the supply and capacity of schools. One-quarter of public schools have no counselors and over half do not have a social worker, yet schools are being asked to deal with more of the health and mental health needs of their students through legislation as well as increasingly identified needs by school staff. As many as 1 in 5 young people have a mental disorder of some kind.[2-4] Mental health difficulties in youth are one of the strongest predictors of academic failure[5] and absenteeism.[1] Despite the high prevalence of mental illness in children and adolescents, 80% of young people with mental illness do not seek help or receive adequate treatment.[6-8] Schools have a key role as places where youth at risk are identified and seek help; in those youth receiving services, 70% report school is the primary source of care.[9]

MENTAL HEALTH LITERACY

Mental health literacy has received attention in terms of reducing stigma, promoting resiliency, and providing education about mental health and mental illness. The objective is to build a knowledge base and provide capacity-building tools for identifying and helping youth with mental illness by targeting health literacy tools for both youth and the adults in their world. The school role in physical health has been recognized for decades as a vehicle for health promotion (eg, the teaching of nutrition through national food guidelines), early identification (eg, vision and hearing tests), and intervention (eg, vaccinations). The potential for schools in dealing with mental health promotion and identification of mental disorders has been identified, but research is lacking as to the outcomes of increasing mental health literacy in terms of prevention of mental health disorders. In terms of changes in attitudes and behaviors, evidence supports that along with education there need to be some practical skills and strategies implemented and that integrated programs are more successful than stand-alone, solo education opportunities.[10,11]

Definitions of health literacy have undergone substantial conceptual development in the past 10 years. Early definitions emphasized "the ability to read and comprehend prescriptions bottles, appointment slips and other essential health-related materials required to successfully function as a patient."[12] Newer definitions have been expanded to include "the degree to which individuals have the capacity to obtain, process, and understand basic health information and services to make appropriate health decisions."[13]

The most important factors affecting knowledge uptake are the level of literacy in general and health literacy in particular of young people. This concept is consistent with current research showing that one of the most important determinants of health is health literacy,[12] which is itself influenced by general literacy levels. A recent systematic review of evidence on literacy and health outcomes concluded that "low literacy is associated with several adverse health outcomes, including low health knowledge, increased incidence of chronic illness, and less than optimal use of preventive health services."[14] Other studies have shown that although young people believe that accurate health information is available, they do not necessarily have the skills to determine the accuracy of the information in order to make an informed decision about their health.[15]

The evolution of the definition of health and mental literacy marks an important change in our understanding of what health literacy encompasses. The definition has expanded from following health instructions to making complex decisions about health, and it encompasses knowledge acquisition theory that learning is shaped by what is already known and how information is known.[16] This decision-making is influenced by a range of educational, cognitive, cultural, and ethical issues including levels of literacy in general.[14,17] The fundamental assumption of most health and mental health programs, irrespective of their intended outcome or delivery mechanism, is that knowledge, skills, and awareness can be acquired and that their acquisition can lead to better health choices and positive health improvement.

Kelly and colleagues[18] recently highlighted the growing body of literature documenting mental health literacy deficits in adolescents and young adults and reviewed a number of health literacy programs. They identified four different types of programs, few of which have been evaluated at all: (1) whole-community campaigns, (2) youth-oriented community campaigns, (3) school-based interventions teaching help-seeking mental health literacy and/or resiliency, and (4) programs designed to train individuals to better intervene in a crisis.[18] For most, the core element of health literacy is decision-making. Some research suggests that young people begin making decisions about their own health from about age 15.[19] Given the strong link between general levels of literacy and health literacy and the evidence that young people begin making decisions about their health during their middle school years, there is a credible argument that health decision-making skills should be an integral part of the school curriculum even before health decisions are being made.[20] Long-term health and well-being of all individuals are inextricably linked with the level of education and literacy that individuals attain over the course of their lifetime.[21]

The focus on application of newly learned skills to make good health choices underscores the difference between knowledge mobilization (knowledge transfer and uptake) and health literacy. Knowledge transfer and knowledge uptake are best viewed as the processes by which health literacy will be achieved. The long-term success of any school-based mental health program or intervention will depend on individuals recognizing appropriate instances to apply skills in new contexts, having the information to make good health choices or knowing where to find this information, and identifying when they need help. Although decision-making is often implied in what many refer to as knowledge transfer, the methods for improving the uptake of facts, increasing the awareness of conditions, and teaching decision-making may be very different. Arguably, it is all three—the uptake of facts, increased awareness, and capacity for decision making—that are required for any type of school-based health initiative to succeed, whether it is a school-based health service, an early detection program, or a universal prevention program. For example, school-based health centers rely on youth seeking help for mental health problems. Help-seeking is a multistep decision that involves (a) identifying a difficulty, (b) acknowledging that the difficulty warrants help or treatment, (c) knowing that treatment is available and effective, (d) deciding that treatment is desired, (e) being motivated to seek treatment, and (f) seeking help.[22–24] Each of these steps can be understood within a health literacy framework; acquiring, integrating, and applying knowledge (decision-making) to increase a certain outcome (improved help-seeking).

Many school-based initiatives present written material in a one-time or noninte-grated format and in didactic fashion. However, more and more evidence shows us that youth do not retain this information or use it to change their attitudes and behaviors.[25] Nor does this delivery method fit with the dynamics of change and new knowledge and research in child and youth mental health.[26,27] *Are we training our youth to be good health consumers, to look after their health, seek help when needed, and make good health decisions?* Education literature shows that learning takes place in an environment that allows exploring and self-direction.[28,29] In looking at the challenges of health literacy, it has been recommended that health curricula integrate the usage of Internet delivery of information to teach the skills necessary for youth to acquire and evaluate health information.[17,30,31] The best chance for knowledge to be used is when it is immediately applicable.[32] By engaging youth in the process of health learning in an interactive, immediate, and individual way, knowledge is more relevant and can be used and integrated in context.

The dissemination of resources on Web sites represents one of the most rapidly growing uses of the Internet in an attempt to increase both knowledge transfer and knowledge uptake (**Box 1**). In terms of knowledge transfer, Web sites that list information sheets (eg, www.health.nih.gov; www.aacap.org), maintain Q&A bulletin boards (eg, www.goaskalice.org), provide screening tools and information (eg, www.beyondblue.org.au, www.downyourdrink.org.uk, www.schoolpsychiatry.org), or document the effectiveness of various interventions and treatments (eg, www. nrepp.samhsa.gov) are numerous. Internet-based mental health resources offer a unique opportunity to link young people and those working with youth with health expert information and tools to help them with health decision-making, identifying needs, and accessing resources.[31,33] However, despite the large number of Web sites and search engines available, a recent study reported that 69% of teens could not find information they were looking for about sex and adolescent sexuality and that 62% found obstacles in getting information online.[34] There is also difficulty assessing the accuracy and applicability of information online.[30,35] The ease with which information can be deployed online is not only a success of the Internet but potentially one of the greatest obstacles facing many online programs. With such a large number of sites and no way for most users to determine the credibility of the information, attracting and retaining users will remain a challenge, and there are little or no data examining the extent to which online health resources work to change knowledge, attitudes, and behaviors. However, the potential benefit in terms of increased availability and accessibility for any type of school-based program or intervention whether school-based health centers, early detection initiatives, specific illness support strategies, or universal school-based programs is considerable.

SCHOOL MENTAL HEALTH RESEARCH

The number of health promotion and prevention initiatives addressing mental health difficulties is rapidly expanding. By the end of 2002, there were estimated to be over 1200 outcome studies on prevention, health promotion, and drug abuse prevention in youth.[36] The New Freedom Commission on Mental Health's *Achieving the Promise: Transforming Mental Health Care in America* emphasized the importance of mental

---

Box 1
School mental health Web sites and resources

○ Massachusetts General Hospital, School Psychiatry resources for parents, educators, and clinicians to support youth with mental health disorders in school.
http://www.massgeneral.org/schoolpsychiatry/

○ Canadian Mental Health Association. High School Curriculum for Mental Health Education. Resources include curriculum, lesson plans, and video clips providing education about mental illness.
http://www.cmha.ca/highschoolcurriculum/

○ University of California, Los Angeles, School Mental Health Project. Clearinghouse of resources for supporting school mental health.
http://smhp.psych.ucla.edu/

○ Australian Mental Health Promotion Site and School Program for Elementary Schools and Secondary Schools. Includes great downloadable resources.
http://www.kidsmatter.edu.au/ (preschool and elementary)
http://www.mindmatters.edu.au (secondary)

○ University of Maryland Center for School Mental Health. Resources for educators, students, families, and clinicians.
http://www.schoolmentalhealth.org/

○ My Health Magazine. Canadian mental health literacy program for secondary schools, youth and educators versions. http://www.myhealthmagazine.net

○ Teen Mental Health site. Canadian resource of mental health information and education programs (including curriculum) for youth, families, clinicians, and educators.
http://teenmentalhealth.org

○ Communities and School Promoting Health. A Canadian School Health Knowledge Network providing links and resources for school health in including mental health.
http://www.safehealthyschools.org

○ Promoting Relationships and Eliminating Violence (PREVNet). A Canadian network of research, community, and nongovernmental organizations with resources for bullying prevention and intervention.
http://prevnet.ca

○ Children's Mental Health Ontario. Resources for teachers and professionals working with youth to address mental health issues and promote mental wellness.
http://www.kidsmentalhealth.ca/professionals/mh_for_teachers_classrooms.php?print=1

○ Centre for Addiction and Mental Health. Resources for teachers and schools.
http://camh.net/education/Resources_teachers_schools/index.html

○ Canadian Psychiatric Research Foundation. *When Something's Wrong* handbooks for families and teachers around common mental health problems in children and adolescents
www.cprf.ca

---

health in learning and social/emotional development of children and youth, recommending improved and expanded school-based mental health services.[37] A number of school-based programs and initiatives have been developed to address broad goals including health promotion, early identification, crisis response, and prevention and treatment of emotional and behavioral disorders.[38,39] These programs may use one or more distinct delivery mechanisms including full-service school-based health centers, screening programs, and classroom and school-based strategies and curricula.[40] The articles in this issue overview some of these programs and the current research and best evidence practices in school mental health. Most programs face system obstacles and methods of delivering service to young people in schools, ranging from the practical challenges in maintaining school-based health centers[41–43] to the implementation and sustainability of evidence-based school-wide programming[44] and the viability of screening programs.[45] Despite the growing number of school-based mental health initiatives, there is no identified best practice model for delivering and sustaining these programs.[40] Direct service models include school-based mental health centers, crisis intervention, school-community mental health center collaborations, and fee-for-service mental health contracts. Indirect service models include school system consultation, prevention and intervention programs, early identification screening programs, Web-based mental health resources, and on-site or video consultation with other mental health clinicians. The model adopted by a school depends on resources, state law, student and school needs and priorities, and the focus of the consultant.

Universal prevention programs address the school system as a whole and aim to better the overall educational climate and learning environment by coordinating community and outside resources. Specific intervention/prevention models target a wide range of risk behaviors including anxiety, depression, substance abuse, and bullying/violence. Evidence examining the effectiveness of whole-school programs suggests that the effectiveness of universal programs (delivered to all students) is modest in addressing specific problems but can have broad impact on school climate and has more success with a focus on developing protective factors than by decreasing negative risk factors. In some cases indicated prevention programs (delivered to students with elevated symptoms) and selected prevention programs (delivered to high-risk students) may be more effective in targeting specific problems.[46]

SUMMARY

Psychiatrists are in a unique position to advocate for school-based mental health supports, whether for the individual or school system as a whole. The importance of mental health literacy and knowledge mobilization tools in health decision-making for youth and the research in school-based mental health interventions provide the background needed for working with schools. Although the general goal of improving health literacy among youth may be easily endorsed, there are competing interests among educators, administrators, and policy makers. Ensuring that the resource, whether Internet-based or school-based, remains of value to multiple stakeholders, even with minimal investment of effort, is essential. Successful school models and interventions, whether they be for the individual or school-wide, integrate the school, family, and community (including clinical) in coordinating services and instituting reform. Common elements in successful intervention and prevention programs include youth being connected to trusted adults, access and coordination of appropriate programs and services with ongoing evaluation, education and training of school staff (building local capacity), cognitive behavioral and skill-based intervention programs integrated within school programs, and longer term multiyear interventions.

The articles in this issue are designed to provide information useful for clinicians in school mental health. The articles include overviews of broad topics in school-based mental health (eg, education legislation, mental health literacy, global school-based mental health, school mental health program sustainability) and more specific disorder-based school mental health areas (eg, depression, anxiety, substance abuse, attention-deficit/hyperactivity disorder, disruptive/conduct behaviors). Psychiatrists and other school-based clinicians can help schools identify and implement appropriate programs or services depending on the needs and resources of the individual and school system. Improving mental health literacy and outcomes among youth will ultimately depend on our collective ability as educators, health professionals, and parents to achieve a daily, sustainable presence in the lives of young people—both in and out of the classroom.

REFERENCES

1. DeSocio J, Hootman J. Children's mental health and school success. J Sch Nurs 2004;20:189–96.
2. Esser G, Schmidt MH, Woerner W. Epidemiology and course of psychiatric disorders in school-age children--results of a longitudinal study. J Child Psychol Psychiatry 1990;31:243–63.
3. Offord DR, Boyle, MH, Szatmari P, et al. Ontario child health study II. Six-month prevalence of disorder and rates of service utilization. Arch Gen Psychiatry 1987;44: 832–6.
4. Roberts RE, Attkisson CC, Rosenblatt A. Prevalence of psychopathology among children and adolescents. Am J Psychiatry 1998;155(6):715–25.
5. Kessler RC, Foster CL, Saunders WB, et al. Social consequences of psychiatric disorders I: Educational attainment. Am J Psychiatry 1995;152:1026–32.
6. Langer TS, Gersten JC, Greene EL, et al. Treatment of psychological disorders among urban children. J Consult Clin Psychol 1974;2:170–9.
7. Leaf PJ, Alegria M, Cohen P, et al. Mental health service use in the community and schools: results from the four-community MECA study. J Am Acad Child Adolesc Psychiatry 1996;35:889–97.
8. National Advisory Mental Health Council. National plan for research on child and adolescent mental disorders. Rockville (MD): US Department of Health and Human Services, Public Health Service, ADAMHA; 1990.
9. US Department of Health and Human Services. Mental health: a report of the Surgeon General. Rockville (MD): US Department of Health and Human Services, Substance Abuse and Mental Health Services Administration, Center for Mental Health Services. http://www.surgeongeneral.gov/library/mentalhealth/home.html. Published 1999. Accessed September 15, 2011.
10. Grimshaw JM, Shirran L, Thomas R, et al. Changing provider behavior: an overview of systematic reviews of interventions. Med Care 2001;39(8 Suppl 2):2–45.
11. Browne G, Gafni A, Roberts J, et al. Effective/efficient mental health programs for school-age children: a synthesis of reviews. Soc Sci Med 2004;58:1367–84.
12. American Medical Association Ad Hoc Committee on Health Literacy. Health literacy: report of the Council on Scientific Affairs. JAMA 1992:281(6):552–7.
13. United States Department of Health and Human Services, Office of Disease Prevention and Health Promotion. Healthy people. Washington, DC: US Department of Health and Human Services; 2000.
14. Rootman I, Ronson B. Literacy and health research in canada: where have we been and where should we go? Can J Public Health 2005;96:S62–77.
15. Skinner H, Biscope S, Poland B, et al. How adolescents use technology for health information: implications for health professionals from focus group studies. J Med Internet Res 2003;5(4):e32.
16. Broner N, Franczak M, Dye C, et al. Knowledge transfer, policy making and community empowerment: a consensus model approach for providing public mental health and substance abuse services. Psychiatr Q 2001;72:79–102.
17. Chiarelli L, Edwards P. Building healthy public policy. Can J Public Health 2006;97: S37–42.

18. Kelly CM, Jorm AF, Wright A. Improving mental health literacy as a strategy to facilitate early intervention for mental disorders. Med J Aust 2007;187:S26–30.
19. Taylor L, Adelman HS, Kaser-Boyd N. Attitudes toward involving minors in decisions. Prof Psychol Res Pr 1984;15:436–49.
20. Gray J, Klein P, Noyce T, et al. The Internet: a window on adolescent health literacy.J Adolesc Health, 2005;37:243.
21. Berkman ND, DeWalt DA, Pignone MP, et al. Literacy and health outcomes. Evidence Report/technology assessment No. 87 (Prepared by RTI International–University of North Carolina Evidence-Based Practice Center under contract No. 290-02-0016). AHRQ publication No. 04-E007-2. Rockville (MD): Agency for Healthcare Research and Quality; January 2004.
22. Santor DA, Kususmakar V, Poulin C, et al. Facilitating help seeking behavior and referrals for mental health difficulties in school aged boys and girls: a school-based intervention. J Youth Adolesc 2006;36:741–52.
23. Santor DA, Poulin C, Leblanc J, et al. Adolescent help seeking behavior on the Internet: opportunities for health promotion and early identification of difficulties. J Am Acad Child Adolesc Psychiatry 2007;46:50–9.
24. Gulliver A, Griffiths KM, Christensen H. Perceived barriers and facilitators to mental health help-seeking in young people: a systematic review. BMC Psychiatry 2010;10: 113.
25. Small S, Memmo M. Contemporary models of youth development and problem prevention: toward an integration of terms, concepts and models. Fam Relat 2004; 53:3–11.
26. Flay BR. Positive youth development requires comprehensive health promotion programs. Am J Health Behav 2002;26:404–24.
27. Elias MJ, Weissberg RP. Primary prevention: educational approaches to enhance social and emotional learning. J Sch Health 2000;70(5):186–90.
28. Bass L, Anderson-Pattton V, Allender J. Self-study as a way of teaching and learning. In: Loughran J, Russell T, editors. Improving teacher education through self-study. London. RoutledgeFalmer; p. 56–70.
29. Albanese MA, Mitchell S. Problem-based learning: a review of literature on its outcomes and implementation issues. Acad Med 1993;68(1):52–81.
30. Gray N, Klein J, Noyce P, et al. Health information seeking behaviour in adolescence. Soc Sci Med 2005;60:1467–78.
31. Santor D, Bagnell A. Enhancing the effectiveness and sustainability of school-based mental health programs: maximizing program participation, knowledge uptake and ongoing evaluation using internet based resources. Advances in School Mental Health Promotion 2008;1:17–28.
32. Jacobson N, Butterill D, Goering P. Consulting as a strategy for knowledge transfer. Milbank Q 2005;83:299–321.
33. Wilson CJ, Bushnell JA, Caputi P. Early access and help seeking: practice implications and new initiatives. Early Interv Psychiatry 2001;5:S34–9.
34. Frappier J, Kaufman M, Baltzer F, et al. Sex and sexual health: a survey of Canadian youth and mothers. Paediatr Child Health 2008;13:25–30.
35. Benigeri M, Pluye P. Shortcomings of health information on the Internet. Health Promot Int 2003;18(4):381–6.
36. Weisz JR, Sandler IN, Durlak JA, et al. Promoting and protecting youth mental health through evidence-based prevention and treatment. Am Psychol 2005;60:628–48.
37. Brener ND, Weist M, Adelman H, et al. Mental health and social services: results from the School Health Policies and Programs Study 2006. J Sch Health 2007;77:486–99.

38. Adelman HS, Taylor L. Mental health in schools and system restructuring. Clin Psychol Rev 1999;19:137–63.
39. Adelman HS, Taylor L. Promoting mental health in schools in the midst of school reform. J Sch Health 2000;70:171.
40. Foster S, Rollefson M, Doksum T, et al. School mental health services in the United States 2002-2003. DHHS Pub. No. (SMA) 05-4068. Rockville (MD): Center for Mental Health Services, Substance Abuse and Mental Health Services Administration. http://www.projectforum.org/docs/SchoolMentalHealthServicesintheUS.pdf. Published 2005. Accessed September 15, 2011.
41. Armbruster P, Lichtman J. Are school based mental health services effective? Evidence from 36 inner city schools. Community Ment Health J 1999;35:493–504.
42. Durlak JA. Primary prevention programs in schools. In: Ollendick TH, Prinz RJ, editors. Advances in clinical child psychology. New York: Plenum Press; 1997; p. 283–318.
43. Weist MD. Expanded school mental health services: a national movement in progress. In: Ollendick TH, Prinz RJ, editors. Advances in clinical child psychology. New York: Plenum; 1997: p. 319–52.
44. Schaeffer CM, Bruns E, Weist M, et al. Overcoming challenges to using evidence based interventions in schools. J Youth Adolesc 2005;34:15–22.
45. Hallfors D, Brodish PH, Khatapoush S, et al. Feasibility of screening adolescents for suicide risk in "real world" high school settings. Am J Public Health 2006;96:282–7.
46. Bagnell A, Bostic J. School consultation. In: Kaplan BJ, Sadock VA, editors. Comprehensive textbook of psychiatry. 9th edition. Philadelphia: Lippincott, Williams and Wilkins; 2009: p. 3850–64.

International School Mental Health: Global Approaches, Global Challenges, and Global Opportunities

Yifeng Wei, Med*, Stan Kutcher, MD, FRCPC, FCAHS

KEYWORDS

- Mental health • Schools • Evidence-based interventions
- Integrated pathway to care • World Health Organizations

COMPLEXITIES OF ADDRESSING SCHOOL MENTAL HEALTH GLOBALLY

Health and education are inextricably related, and play a fundamental role in the development of children and youth. Young people cannot learn effectively if their health is poor, so health literacy is important in enhancing health, leading to a wide variety of school health programs being implemented globally.

School health programs have evolved increasingly from physical health only to include mental health interventions. Three distinct, overlapping phases have occurred. Phase 1 identified the important role of schools in providing immunizations and health screening for selected health problems (eg, vision, hearing, scoliosis), providing health essentials (eg, food programs, safe water and sanitation services), and preventing of communicable diseases and injuries.[1,2] Phase 2 evolved primarily over the past 20 years, as social and emotional health and well-being have been added. Specifically, the promotion of safe and emotionally healthy school environments, life skills education, prevention of substance abuse and violence/aggression, and detection of learning disabilities have been added.[1,2] More recently, mental health and mental illness are areas of intense focus in schools, including the importance of promoting positive mental health through education, and the early identification/prevention of mental disorders.[2,3] This third phase of school health framework has become an important area of innovation and research.[4]

Addressing mental health in schools varies substantially across the globe depending on diverse variables such as social norms, accessibility of mental health care, socioeconomic status, religion, culture, geographic location. In countries embroiled in war or where human rights and law enforcement are weak or nonexistent, many

IWK Health Centre, 5850 University Avenue, PO Box 9700, Halifax, Nova Scotia, Canada B3K 6R8
* Corresponding author.
E-mail address: Yifeng.Wei@iwk.nshealth.ca

Child Adolesc Psychiatric Clin N Am 21 (2012) 11–27
doi:10.1016/j.chc.2011.09.005
1056-4993/12/$ – see front matter © 2012 Elsevier Inc. All rights reserved.

schools may not function consistently, and basic needs such as safety, shelter, and security may not be present. The impetus for initiating school-based health programs has sometimes been to target a specific public health issue such as the prevention of communicable disease (eg, HIV/AIDS in Zimbabwe and Thailand), or the prevention of teen pregnancy (eg, in Mexico and the Caribbean). In some other regions, faith-based or religious education predominates, and how this relates to school mental health programs has not been well studied. Moreover, even within a jurisdiction substantive differences between various schools may make a single model approach to school mental health unworkable, although common policy and evaluation frameworks may be necessary to direct programs and activities.[5]

These realities all impact the conceptualization, development, and implementation of school mental health initiatives and illustrate how local and contextual factors play important roles as school mental health approaches are developed. What constitutes a school mental health priority in 1 area may be vastly different from the priorities in another. This recognition of the global reality suggests that the development of school mental health approaches should be driven by specific population needs, contextualized to fit local realities, and link mental health to physical health and learning outcomes. All stakeholders should be aware of these complexities so that they are able to develop and implement appropriate, yet feasible, policies, plans and programs to respond to mental health priorities of children and adolescents within the school setting.

DEVELOPMENT OF GLOBAL SCHOOL MENTAL HEALTH INITIATIVES

Internationally, early interest in school mental health was led by United Nations Agencies, such as the World Health Organization (WHO), the United Nations Children's Fund, and the United Nations Educational, Scientific and Cultural Organization (UNESCO). In 1994, the WHO developed a school mental health model promoting mental health and included mental health education addressing knowledge, attitudes, and behaviors, and the prevention and treatment of psychosocial problems and mental disorders.[3] To develop such programs, the establishment of collaborative teams involving the family, educators, mental health professionals, and the wider community; the assessment of the school environment; development of a plan; monitoring and evaluation; and program review and modification were advocated.[3] Components of this model have been integrated into a number of school health initiatives, such as the Health Promoting Schools approach, to address various aspects of mental health (eg, substance abuse, antisocial behavior, depression/suicide, self-esteem, safe and socially supportive school environments).[6] More than 40 countries have applied these Health Promoting School approaches and preliminary studies have demonstrated evidence of promising effectiveness for some of these initiatives.[6]

UNESCO has also supported the advancement of mental health in schools through its global Education For All movement. The Education For All movement has identified education as a fundamental human right for all, including those with mental disabilities. It further required attention to mental health and emotional support as a learning enabler.[7] Programs endorsed by UNESCO have generally focused on facilitating safe and socially supportive school environments by addressing topics such as bullying, violence, interpersonal conflicts, and life skills education in the school setting.[8]

Recently, international interest in school mental health has been further developed through non-United Nation's approaches, such as through the establishment of the International Alliance for Child and Adolescent Mental Health and Schools.[9] This organization spans more than 30 countries and aims to promote mental health via a whole-school approach encompassing mental health promotion, prevention and intervention. It has built-in communication mechanisms for its members, and supported interdisciplinary approaches and collaborations (www.intercamhs.org). Other global non-United Nations organizations, such as the World Psychiatric Association, the International Association for Child and Adolescent Psychiatry and Allied Professions,[10] and the Clifford Beers Foundation have also recognized the importance of addressing child and youth mental health in schools and funded various mental health programs. The Presidential World Psychiatric Association Program on child mental health[11] and the creation of peer-reviewed publications such as *School Mental Health* (Springer) and *Advances in School Mental Health Promotion* (Clifford Beers Foundation) have additionally stimulated global attention in this area.

SCHOOL MENTAL HEALTH AT THE NATIONAL/COUNTRY LEVEL

A number of developed countries, including the United States, Canada, Australia, New Zealand, and many European nations have taken initiatives to address school mental health nationally. In the United States, the President's New Freedom Commission Report[12] regarded expanding and improving school mental health programs as a federal commitment. A number of nationally active school mental health centers have received federal funding to advance school mental health practice and research. The Centers for Disease Control and Prevention's Division of Adolescent and School Health has proposed a coordinated school health framework that centers around 8 critical and interrelated components, including the integration of mental health and services in schools (available at: http://www.cdc.gov/healthyyouth/cshp/index.htm). The US Department of Education has provided financial and infrastructure support to increase student access to quality mental health care through programs that link school systems with local mental health service systems (available at: http://www2.ed.gov/programs/mentalhealth/index.html). With the support of government agencies and researchers, numerous school mental health programs have been created, such as the Massachusetts General Hospital school psychiatry website (available at: www.schoolpsychiatry.org). Many of these programs have traditionally focused on the treatment of mental disorders in individuals; however, in recent years, increasing attention has been paid to address issues of mental health promotion and prevention.[13]

In Canada, the Mental Health Commission of Canada has recently developed a national child and youth mental health framework, titled "Evergreen,"[14] that has identified schools as a key venue for addressing child and youth mental health. This national child and youth mental health framework raises public awareness, provides support to provinces and territories as they create their policies and plans, and serves as a resource base. The Province of Ontario, in its recently released child and youth mental health strategy, has identified a number of initiatives addressing mental health and schools.[15] School mental health initiatives have been developed nationally and regionally in Canada to address child and youth mental health needs in schools. These include the Mental Health Identification and Navigation: A School-Based Integrated Pathway to Care Model,[16] which addresses youth mental health through an integrated and flexible model that brings together mental health promotion; early identification, prevention, and intervention; and coordinated community-based continuing care. Mental health literacy has been highlighted as a foundational component in the school mental health field and a priority.[17] Mental health literacy programs, such as the Mental Health and High School Curriculum Guide (available at: http://teenmentalhealth.org/index.php/curriculum/)[16] and the *MyHealth Magazine* (available at: http://www.myhealth.yoomagazine.net/)[18] are 2 nationally available examples of programs designed to improve the understanding of mental health and mental illness for children, youth, and educators.

In Australia, the Council of Australian Governments' national action plan highlighted schools as the starting point to shape research and practice in school mental health.[19] Innovations have included the adoption of the WHO Health Promoting Schools model and the whole school involvement approach. KidsMatter is a national primary (elementary) school mental health promotion, prevention, and early intervention initiative (available at: http://www.kidsmatter.edu.au/), and there is a similar national program for secondary schools, MindMatters (available at: http://www.mindmatters. edu.au/default.asp).[20] MindMatters has been adopted widely in Australia and in other parts of the world. Beyondblue is a government-funded initiative, developed as a national resource and research program to address domains associated with depression, anxiety, and related substance misuse disorders in Australia (available at: http://www.beyondblue.org.au/index.aspx).[21] Under the Beyondblue framework, many school programs, such as the "ybblue" youth program, "Tackling Depression in Schools," and the "Schools Research Initiative Report," have been disseminated to schools.

In the United Kingdom, there have also been a number of recent developments in advancing school mental health. For example, the Departments of Health and Education have promoted mental health in schools to enhance educational and social outcomes.[22-24] The Department for Education has promoted the Social and Emotional Aspects of Learning program. The Social and Emotional Aspects of Learning is "a comprehensive, whole-school approach to promoting the social and emotional skills that are thought to underpin effective learning, positive behavior, regular attendance, staff effectiveness and the emotional health and well-being of all who learn and work in schools."[25] A recent National Strategies Report indicates that Social and Emotional Aspects of Learning is currently implemented in about 90% of primary schools and 70% of secondary schools in the United Kingdom.[26] Another national program funded by the Department for Children, Schools and Families is the Targeted Mental Health in School Project delivered to children aged 5 to 13, with the intent to improve their mental well-being and assist them in addressing mental health problems more quickly. The ideological foundation of the Targeted Mental Health in School Project model asserts that the success of school mental health programs resides in the strategic integration of all related stakeholders to deliver "flexible, responsive and effective early intervention mental health services for children and young people," and recognizes the importance of evidence-informed practice that can be tailored to meet local needs.[27]

In Europe, the European Commission has launched the European Pact for Mental Health and Well-being listing mental health education in youth as 1 of its 5 priority areas.[28] It urges the integration of mental health education into curricula and extracurricular activities, and the provision of mental health training for professionals in education, health, and other related agencies.[28] Many school mental health programs are linked through the European Network of Health Promoting Schools with its over 40 member nations. A mental health promotion training program was created for teachers and others working with young people within European Network of Health Promoting Schools.[29] The program teaches professionals working in school settings practical steps to improve the mental and emotional health of youth.

Despite the increasing attention on school mental health in many developed countries, activities in developing countries lag far behind. Many developing countries do not have a child and youth mental health policy, or the resources and capacity to address mental health in children and youth. This reality has encouraged a number of international organizations to take leadership in exploring pathways to promote mental health in schools in some middle to low income countries.

A recent collaborative effort is the establishment of a Child Mental Health Awareness Task Force between the World Psychiatric Association, the WHO, and the International Association for Child and Adolescent Psychiatry and Allied Professions.[10,30] The task force developed a resource manual to promote child mental health awareness worldwide. This mental health education resource was introduced in nine countries for implementation in high school classrooms delivered to approximately 3600 students, teachers and parents in Armenia, Azerbaijan, Brazil, China, Egypt, Georgia, Israel, Russia, and Uganda.[30] Other developing countries in the Asia–Pacific region and South Africa have addressed child and youth mental health needs through health-promoting school initiatives.[6,31,32] These interventions have provided important lessons about the feasibility of developing and implementing school mental health education programs in such a wide range of environments. Unfortunately, the impact of these initiatives on mental health outcomes is not yet known. In many middle- or low-income countries the political interest in, the priority of, or the funding capacity for, child and youth mental health remains problematic.

EVIDENCE FOR SCHOOL MENTAL HEALTH INTERVENTIONS

The emerging field of school mental health has attracted researchers from around the globe to clarify the effectiveness of these programs. Effective, safe, and cost-effective (ESCe) school mental health interventions are essential for global dissemination of programming and funding from governments, international agencies, and other third-party donors. In resource-challenged countries, investment in non–evidence-based programs is not likely to receive funding priority. Even in developed countries, policy makers and third-party funders are demanding evidence of ESCe before widespread implementation of programs. Program developers, policy makers, and providers must show that well-meaning interventions meet independently determined ESCe criteria, and that both research and practice frameworks can be developed both nationally and globally that effectively address this need.

Table 1 is a brief synthesis (using a review of reviews methodology) of findings from the most recent systematic reviews (1995–2011)[33-52] for the effectiveness of school mental health programs for mental health promotion, prevention/early identification, and intervention. These programs cover a wide spectrum of mental health topics, including the promotion of pro-social skills and social/emotional well-being, stigma toward mental illness, violence and aggressive behaviors, substance abuse/misuse, depression, suicide, anxiety, and eating disorders. The reviews cover programs with research evidence globally, but at present studies are limited to developed countries, with most of the research emanating from the United States, Australia, United Kingdom, and Canada.

Two systematic reviews[33,34] of pro-social and social/emotional well-being school interventions have identified the potential value of such school based mental health promotion programs, especially those utilizing a whole school approach involving students, educators, families, and the wider community. One review[35] of school programs designed to reduce stigma toward mental illness suggests some evidence that mental health curricula designed to educate children and youth about stigma toward mental illness may be beneficial in positively changing students' attitudes and behavior (at least in the short term). Five reviews have addressed the issue of school-based interventions to reduce violence and aggressive behaviors in children and youth.[36-40] These reviews included universal, selective, and targeted school-based programs from the elementary to high school ages. Reductions in aggressive

Table 1
Evidence for the effectiveness of school mental health interventions: A summary of systematic reviews

Intervention domains	Review Reference	Outcome Measurement	Intervention Type and Participants Age	Intervention Strategies	Effectiveness	Level of Evidence[a]	CE	Program Safety
Promotion/ Pro-social	Lister-Sharp et al (1999); 24 Studies from US (18), UK (3), Australia (1), and Israel (2) Wells et al (2003); 17 studies from US (16), and Israel (1)	Self-esteem; self-efficacy; positive relationship; empathy; coping skills; stress management; life skills; bullying and aggression; suicide	Universal age: mostly elementary school student, as well as middle and high school students	Using whole-school approach that include school ethos, curriculum and involvement of the family and community; delivered as curriculum mainly by mental health professionals	Short-term positive findings identified in areas including: self-esteem, stress management, life skills, personal responsibility and rights, bullying and aggression, coping skills (girls), empathy (girls), hopelessness (girls); negative findings identified in areas of coping skills and hopelessness in boys; mixed finding in suicide programs. No effects identified in areas of empathy in boys; positive short-term finding identified in whole school approach as opposed to brief, class-based programs	Weak (Lister-Sharp et al, 1999); Unclear (Wells et al, 2003)	Insufficient data for CE	Negative safety findings in coping skills and hopelessness in boys

		Mental health knowledge; attitudes; help-seeking behaviors	Intervention type NR. Age: mostly high school students	Education-only interventions; contact-only interventions; education and contact interventions	Unable to determine what specific program components work owing to significant design and methodologic limitations of included studies; mental health curriculum may be a beneficial approach	Weak	NR	NR
Stigma	Schachter, et al, (2008); 40 studies (study country NR)							
Violence/ aggression	Hahn, et al, (2007); 69 studies from high-income countries Mytton, et al, (2002); 44 studies from US (39), Canada (4) and Australia (1) Mytton, et al, (2006); 56 studies from US (43), Canada (5), Argentina (2) and Australia (1) Schecknerk, et al, 2002; 16 studies (Study country NR) Wilson & Lipsey, 2003; 221 studies (study country NR)	General violence; antisocial behaviors; bullying; gang activities	Universal; selective; indicated Age: mostly elementary and middle school students, as well as kindergarten and high school students	Cognitive and behavior interventions; social skills enhancement; school/ classroom environmental change; peer mediation	Positive short-term findings in universal interventions in all intervention strategies. Short-term reduction in aggression identified in secondary prevention (effect size, −0.36; 95% CI, −0.54 to −0.19; Mytton et al, 2002. Standardized mean difference = −0.41; 95%, −0.56 to −0.26 (Mytton et al, 2006). Reduced aggression most notable in high-risk youth	Unclear level of evidence because of the inclusion of studies of both poor and strong quality (Hahn et al, 2007); weak (Mytton et al, 2009; Schecknerk et al, 2002); NR (Mytton et al, 2002)	NR	NR

(continued on next page)

Table 1
(continued)

Intervention domains	Review Reference	Outcome Measurement	Intervention Type and Participants Age	Intervention Strategies	Effectiveness	Level of Evidence[a]	CE	Program Safety
Depression	Calear & Christensen, 2010; 42 studies (Study country NR) Merry et al, 2009; 21 studies from US (11), Australia (6), China (1), NR (3) Neil & Christensen, 2007; 24 studies from Australia Waddell et al, 2007; 4 studies from US and Australia	Depressive symptoms	Universal; Selective; Indicated Age: children and adolescents (5–19 years)	Cognitive and Behavioral Therapy (CBT); Psychoeducation; Interpersonal Therapy (IPT)	Indicated programs with CBT found most effective in short term; No evidence of effectiveness found in universal programs	Weak (Merry et al, 2004; Neil & Christensen, 2007) Moderate (Waddell et al, 2007); NR (Calear & Christensen, 2010;)	NR	NR

| Anxiety | Neil & Christensen 2007; 24 studies from Australia Neil & Christensen 2009; 27 studies (study country NR) | Symptoms of anxiety | Universal; selective; indicated Age: 9–17 years | CBT; psychoeducation; IPT | Short-term effectiveness for universal and indicated programs with small and moderated effects (effect sizes Cohen d: 0.11–1.37). Both short- and long-term effectiveness with small and moderate effects (effect sizes Cohen d: 0.24–1.36) | Weak | NR | NR |
| Substance abuse | Faggiano et al, 2008; 32 studies from US (30), Canada (1), and Australia (1) Tobler et al, 2000; 207 studies (study country NR) White & Pitts, 1998; 71 studies from US (90% of included studies) | Personal/social skills; knowledge and attitudes; drug/ smoking/ alcohol use prevention | Universal; selective; indicated Age: primary and secondary school students | Interactive/ noninteractive intervention administered by teachers, professionals or peers; drug education by teachers, professionals, or peers | Limited evidence of effectiveness found in small-scale programs ranged from very small to small (Cohen d: 0.15–0.34) in drug knowledge and attitudes, and social skills (Tobler et al, 2000); Limited evidence found in programs for drug prevention in only 2 studies with strong short-term effects, other studies with very small effects (White & Pitts, 1998). Programs developing personal social skills were the most effective for drug prevention in the short term (Faggiano et al, 2008). | Weak (Tobler et al, 2000); weak to moderate (Faggiano et al, 2008); half of included studies were methodologically sound (White & Pitts, 1998) | NR | NR |

(continued on next page)

Table 1
(continued)

Intervention domains	Review Reference	Outcome Measurement	Intervention Type and Participants Age	Intervention Strategies	Effectiveness	Level of Evidence[a]	CE	Program Safety
Suicide	Mann et al, 2005; 2 systematic reviews and 5 studies (study country NR) Robinson et al, 2011; 21 studies (Study country NR)	Suicide attempt, suicide ideation, suicide behavior	Universal; selective Age: adolescents	Curriculum-based education; CBT; group therapy	Very limited evidence of programs in preventing suicidal behaviors, decreasing suicide attempt, deliberate self-harm, or suicidal ideation; only individual CBT-based intervention showed some promising evidence of effectiveness; harmful effects found in some programs	High level of evidence (Oxford level of evidence: 1B and 2A[b]; Mann et al, 2005); unclear due to poor reporting of study design	NR	Harmful effects in some interventions

						CE	Level of evidence	Harm
Eating disorders	Grave, 2003; 29 studies from US (21), Australia (3), UK (2), Canada (1), Switzerland (1), Italy (1); Israel (1) Pratt & Woolfenden, 2009; 12 studies from US (3), Canada (1), Australia (1), Italy (1), NR (6)	Eating attitudes and behaviors; formal diagnosis of eating disorders; general psychological and physical well-being; body mass index; protective psychological factors	Universal; selective Age: 10–20 years	Interactive approach; curriculum-based education; interventions building self-esteem; media presentation and literacy	No evidence of harm for school-based eating disorder programs; evidence of knowledge acquisition; however, no associated change in attitudes and behaviors. Selective programs were more effective than universal programs in behavior change; programs using interactive approaches were more beneficial than traditional didactic methods.	NR	NR (Grave, 2003); high quality of evidence (Pratt & Woolfenden, 2009)	No harm

CE, cost effectiveness; NR, not reported.

[a] Level of evidence was generally decided by review authors by assessing risk of bias in five areas with various tools, including selection, attrition, confounding, outcome measurement, and reporting

[b] Oxford Centre for Evidence Based Medicine, levels of evidence: 1A, systematic reviews of randomized controlled trials (RCTs); 1B, individual RCT; 2A, systematic reviews of cohort studies; 2B, cohort studies, low quality RCTs; 2C, ecological studies; 3A, systematic reviews of case-control studies; 3B, individual case-control study; 4, case-series, poor quality cohort and case-control studies.

behavior were more evident in high-risk youth across most studies, but universal programs were found to have a positive although more modest effect in the overall school environment. Programs that integrated multiple settings (home, school, community) with primary prevention and skills-building (cognitive behavioral strategies and social skills enhancement) approaches had the strongest evidence of effectiveness across age ranges and studies. Reviews of the effectiveness of programs to reduce depression symptoms in children and youth[41,42,44] include universal prevention programs and those programs targeting youth at risk. Universal programs including education and cognitive–behavioral therapy (CBT) skills do not overall show evidence of preventing depression. There is some evidence that selected and indicated programs based on evidence based clinical approaches (CBT and interpersonal therapy) have some impact in reducing depression symptoms in the short term. Evidence of prevention of anxiety programs was presented in 2 recent systematic reviews[43,45] of 30 programs (universal, selective, and indicative) that were mostly CBT as well as psychoeducation, relaxation, and modeling. They found that most of the universal and indicated programs were effective in reducing symptoms of anxiety in the short term and several studies in Australia (FRIENDS program) show some long-term effectiveness as well. Substance abuse/misuse interventions were examined in 3 reviews,[46-48] including universal and selective programs usually targeting late elementary and early adolescence ages. Although drug education had an impact on knowledge, the programs developing personal social skills were found to be the most effective type of school-based intervention in the prevention of early drug use. Evidence for effective suicide prevention programs in the school setting is very limited based on 2 recent systematic reviews.[49,50] Although some curriculum-based programs have improved knowledge and attitudes toward mental illness, very few such programs were evident in preventing suicidal behaviors or had demonstrated program safety. Results suggested only individual CBT-based intervention showed some promising evidence of effectiveness. Two recent, systematic reviews have addressed the prevention of eating disorders.[51,52] In summarizing the findings from more than 40 studies, there was no evidence of harm for school-based eating disorder programs. Targeted/selective programs were more effective than universal programs in behavior change. In addition, programs using interactive approaches were more beneficial than traditional didactic methods. Finally, media literacy and advocacy have a positive impact on changing societal body image ideal.

In summary, there is little substantive evidence to demonstrate the ESCe of many of these initiatives. The quality of research is inconsistent, the relationship between short time changes in these indicators and long-term functional outcome have not been defined, and their safety and cost effectiveness have not been established. Harmful effects were identified in some universal suicide interventions and promotional programs addressing coping skills and hopelessness, especially in boys.[33,49] Universal (delivered to whole school or population) school-based mental health program approaches addressing specific areas such as stigma, suicide, or the prevention of specific disorders (eg, depression, anxiety, substance misuse/abuse, eating disorders) have shown relatively disappointing results to date. There is slightly more evidence for selective (population at risk of a disorder) and indicated/targeted (population with symptoms of disorder) interventions in some areas. Current evidence suggests universal programs may work better for mental health promotion; universal and selective programs may have a role in addressing violent and aggressive behaviors; selective and indicated/targeted programs may elicit better results for prevention of depression and anxiety and eating disorders may show greater response to selective programs. For intervention strategies, the modification or application of clinically derived, evidence-based psychosocial interventions such as CBT were more promising in preventing anxiety, depression, eating disorders, and violent and aggressive behaviors. Substance abuse and violent/aggressive behaviors show more improvement with personal and social skills-building approaches in children and youth. The whole school approach to improving school climate and positive behaviors shows some evidence of reducing violence and aggression in the school setting and improving some indicators of mental health.

Overall, although school-based mental health promotion programs may be promising in promoting mental health or reducing certain risk factors, insufficient evidence currently exists to support these approaches (including their contextualization and modification) globally. Because most of the studies were implemented in developed countries, with relatively similar cultures, the potential for generalizing these programs to other countries has yet to be demonstrated. The wide variety of different health systems, social, economic, and cultural realities that impact ESCe may lead researchers to redesign how to apply such programs, compromising program fidelity in to provide frameworks and components customized to meet local needs and realities. Mental health literacy built on the wider concept of health literacy shows some promise of effectiveness across many different domains, including knowledge acquisition, stigma reduction, and enhanced health-seeking behavior.[20,21]

RECOMMENDATIONS

Schools have been identified as an important venue for health promotion and prevention since the 1950s. The integration of mental health into school health interventions has become an emerging trend for the last 2 decades with substantial increases in developed countries over the last 10 years. Based on the lessons learned to date, the following points may need to be considered and highlighted in future school mental health practice and research.

First, the mental health of children and youth may be most parsimoniously achieved through an integrated and comprehensive "pathway to care" framework that establishes a continuum of child and youth mental health promotion, prevention/early identification, intervention, and continuing care, with the school built in as part of this pathway. Although there is evidence of some empirically based mental health promotion, prevention, and intervention school-based programs, there is very limited information regarding long-term outcomes and sustainability. The pathway to care framework must be developed in such a way as to be both comprehensive and flexible, adaptable to myriad local realities that define both health and education, with school mental health integrated as part of this approach.[16]

Second, mental health literacy should be considered as a foundation for school mental health for all stakeholders involved (eg, students, teachers, parents, student service providers, primary care health providers). A mental health curriculum can be a starting point to facilitate the understanding of mental health and mental illness, change attitudes toward mental illness, and encourage help-seeking behaviors for children and youth. This type of approach should embed mental health education into usual school learning paradigms to enhance knowledge acquisition and address attitudinal and behavioral modifications within an already acceptable mode of delivery. Educators, with appropriate knowledge and training, may be more likely to promote mental health in their everyday activities, identify children and youth at risk for mental health problems, and work more collaboratively with families and health care providers.

Third, more than half of school mental health research reports originate currently from the United States, and many school mental health models have been developed specific to this setting, and not necessarily applicable to other countries. It is essential that other countries with different education and health systems invest more in the development and evaluation of school mental health policies and programs, make those evaluations known globally, and for countries to both network and share their findings through a global network where the most effective components can be identified and extrapolated to diverse environments.

Fourth. the development and independent testing of various school mental health approaches will increase credibility and visibility of global mental health programs. Linking research expertise across countries at different levels of development can accelerate research competency development . Such research capacity building will enhance the quality of existing school mental health research as well as provide support needed for developing countries to move the school mental health agenda forward in their countries.

Finally, school mental health requires global funding priority. At this time, the vast majority of global health and health-related development funding does not go to mental health. Both national development agencies and large international donors need to be engaged in the development and application of school mental health initiatives. For this to occur, a strong global school mental health database, demonstrating the effectiveness, safety, and cost effectiveness of various school mental health initiatives needs to be created and publicized.

SUMMARY

School mental health programs have increasingly been developed over the past decade in a number of developed countries. Examples from these countries demonstrate that both the practice of and research into school mental health are becoming more important to policy makers, educators, health providers, parents, and other stakeholders. Some United Nations agencies (eg, WHO, UNESCO) and other international organizations (eg, International Alliance for Child and Adolescent Mental Health and Schools) have begun work to advance school mental health internationally. Much of this work has focused on mental health promotion, prevention, and on-site or linked identification/triage and intervention programs. Meanwhile, numerous universal, selective, and targeted programs have been developed and applied. School-based mental health programming needs to be considered as part of usual child and youth mental health policies and plans, whether those are national or other jurisdictional (such as state or provincial) in nature. Currently, a paucity of child and youth global mental health policies exist, limiting school-based mental health programs being developed, implemented, or sustained. Mental health in the school setting is shifting to a more complex perspective embracing the importance of including school mental health as part of an integrated continuum of child and youth health.

REFERENCES

1. WHO Expert Committee on Comprehensive School Health Education and Promotion. Promoting health through schools report of a WHO Expert Committee on Comprehensive School Health Education and Promotion. 1997;870. Available at: http://whqlibdoc.who.int/trs/WHO_TRS_870.pdf. Accessed August 27, 2011.
2. World Health Organization. Strategic directions for improving the health and development of children and adolescents. 2003. Available at: http://whqlibdoc.who.int/publications/2003/9241591064.pdf. Accessed August 27, 2011.

3. Hendren R, Weisen R, Birrell OJ. Mental health programmes in schools. 1994. Available at: http://whqlibdoc.who.int/hq/1993/WHO_MNH_PSF_93.3_Rev.1.pdf. Accessed August 27, 2011.

4. Weist M, Evans S, Lever N, editors. Handbook of school mental health: advancing practice and research. Springer: New York; 2003.

5. Price OA, Lear JG. School mental health services for the 21st century: Lessons from the District of Columbia school mental health program. 2008. Available at: http://community.rwjf.org/docs/DOC-1642. Accessed August 27, 2011.

6. Stewart S. What is the evidence of school health promotion in improving health, or preventing disease and, specifically, what is the effectiveness of health promoting schools approach? Copenhagen: WHO Regional Office for Europe; 2006. Available at: http://www.euro.who.int/__data/assets/pdf_file/0007/74653/E88185.pdf. Accessed August 27, 2011.

7. United Nations Educational, Scientific and Cultural Organization. World declaration on education for all and framework for action to meet basic learning needs. 1990. Available at: http://www.unesco.org/education/pdf/JOMTIE_E.PDF. Accessed August 27, 2011.

8. United Nations Educational, Scientific and Cultural Organization. A compendium of good practices of National Commissions for UNESCO. 2004. Available at: http://unesdoc.unesco.org/images/0013/001354/135478e.pdf. Accessed August 27, 2011.

9. Rowling L, Weist M. Promoting the growth, improvement and sustainability of school mental health programs worldwide. Int J Mental Health Promot 2004;6(2):3–11.

10. World Psychiatric Association, World Health Organization, The International Association for Child and Adolescent Psychiatry and Allied Professions. Global child mental health. 2004. Available at: http://www.wpanet.org/globalchild.pdf. Accessed August 27, 2011.

11. Okasha A. The Presidential WPA Program on Child Mental Health. World Psychiatry 2003;2:129–30.

12. New Freedom Commission on Mental Health. Achieving the promise: transforming mental health care in America. Final report. 2003;No. DHHS Pub. SMA-03-3832. Available at: http://store.samhsa.gov/product/Achieving-the-Promise-Transforming-Mental-Health-Care-in-America-Executive-Summary/SMA03-3831. Accessed August 27, 2011.

13. Weist MD, Rowling L. International efforts to advance mental health in schools. Int J Mental Health Promot 2002;4(4):3.

14. Kutcher SP, McLuckie A; for the Child and Youth Advisory Committee, Mental Health Commission of Canada. Evergreen: A child and youth mental health framework for Canada. Calgary, Alberta (Canada): Mental Health Commission of Canada; 2010.

15. Ontario Ministry of Health and Long-Term Care. Open minds, healthy Minds. 2011. Available at: http://www.health.gov.on.ca/english/public/pub/mental/pdf/open_minds_healthy_minds_en.pdf. Accessed August 27, 2011.

16. Wei Y, Kutcher S, Szumilas M. Comprehensive school mental health: an integrated pathway to care model for Canadian secondary schools. McGill J Educ, in press.

17. Santor D, Short K, Ferguson B. Taking mental health to school: a policy-oriented paper on school-based mental health for Ontario. 2009. Available at: http://www.excellenceforchildandyouth.ca/sites/default/files/position_sbmh.pdf. Accessed August 27, 2011.

18. Santor D, Bagnell A. Enhancing the effectiveness and sustainability of school based mental health programs: maximizing program participation, knowledge Uptake and ongoing evaluation using Internet based resources. Adv School Mental Health Promot 2008;1:17–28.
19. Council of Australian Government. National action plan mental health 2006–2011. 2006. Available at: http://www.coag.gov.au/coag_meeting_outcomes/2006-07-14/docs/nap_mental_health.pdf. Accessed August 27, 2011.
20. Anderson S, Doyle M. Student and staff mental health literacy and MindMatters Plus. Australian Journal of Guidance & Counselling 2005;15:209–13.
21. Sawyer MG, Harchak TF, Spence SH, et al. School-based prevention of depression: a 2-year follow-up of a randomized controlled trial of the BeyondBlue schools research initiative. J Adolesc Health 2010;47:297–304.
22. Department of Education and Employment, UK (DfEE). National Healthy School Standard. 1999. Available at: http://www.nice.org.uk/nicemedia/documents/nhss_workingtogether.pdf. Accessed August 27, 2011.
23. Department for Education and Skills, UK (DfES). Promoting children's mental health within early years and school settings. 2001. Available at: https://www.education.gov.uk/publications/eOrderingDownload/0619-2001.pdf. Accessed August 27, 2011.
24. Department of Health, UK (DoH). Saving lives: our healthier nation white paper and reducing health inequalities. 1999. Available at: http://www.dh.gov.uk/prod_consum_dh/groups/dh_digitalassets/@dh/en/documents/digitalasset/dh_4012011.pdf. Accessed August 27, 2011.
25. Department for Children, Schools and Families (UK). Social and emotional aspects of learning for secondary schools. Nottingham: DCSF Publications; 2007.
26. Department for Education, UK (DFE). Social and emotional aspects of learning (SEAL) programme in secondary schools: national evaluation. 2010. Available at: https://www.education.gov.uk/publications/eOrderingDownload/DFE-RB049.pdf. Accessed August 27, 2011.
27. Department for children, schools and families (UK). Targeted mental health in schools project. Using the evidence to inform your approach: a practical guide for headteachers and commissioners. 2008. Available at: https://www.education.gov.uk/publications/eOrderingDownload/00784-2008BKT-EN.pdf. Accessed August 27, 2011.
28. World Health Organization Regional Office for Europe. European PACT for mental health and well-being: EU high-level conference. 2008. Available at: http://ec.europa.eu/health/ph_determinants/life_style/mental/docs/pact_en.pdf. Accessed August 27, 2011.
29. Weare K, Gray G; for the World Health Organization Regional Office for Europe. Promoting mental and emotional health in the European network of Health Promoting Schools: a training manual for teachers and others working with young people. 1995. Available at: http://www.schoolsforhealth.eu/upload/PromotingmentalandemotionalhealthintheENHPS.pdf. Accessed August 27, 2011.
30. Hoven CW, Doan T, Musa GJ, et al. Worldwide child and adolescent mental health begins with awareness: a preliminary assessment in nine countries. Int Rev Psychiatry 2008;20:261–70.
31. Rowling L, Ritchie J. Health promoting schools: issues and future directions for Australia and the Asia Pacific Region. Asia Pac J Public Health 1996;9:33–7.
32. Swart D, Reddy P. Establishing networks for health promoting schools in South Africa. J Sch Health 1999;69(2):47–50.
33. Lister-Sharp D, Chapman S, Stewart-Brown S, et al. Health promoting schools and health promotion in schools: two systematic reviews. Health Technol Assess 1999; 3(22):1–207.

34. Wells J, Barlow J, Stewart-Brown S. A systematic review of universal approaches to mental health promotion in schools. Health Educ 2003;103:197–220.
35. Schachter HM, Girardi A, Ly M, et al. Effects of school-based interventions on mental health stigmatization: a systematic review. Child Adolesc Psychiatry Ment Health 2008;2:18.
36. Hahn R, Fuqua-Whitley D, Wethington H, et al. Effectiveness of universal school-based programs to prevent violent and aggressive behavior: a systematic review. Am J Prev Med 2007;33(Suppl 2):S114–29.
37. Mytton JA, DiGuiseppi C, Gough DA, et al. School-based violence prevention programs: systematic review of secondary prevention trials. Arch Pediatr Adolesc Med 2002;156:752–62.
38. Mytton J, DiGuiseppi C, Gough D, et al. School-based secondary prevention programmes for preventing violence. Cochrane Database Syst Rev 2006;3:CD004606.
39. Scheckner S, Rollin S, Kaiser-Ulrey C, et al. School violence in children and adolescents. J School Violence 2002;1(2):5–32.
40. Wilson SJ, Lipsey MW, Derzon JH. The effects of school-based intervention programs on aggressive behavior: a meta-analysis. J Consult Clin Psychol 2003;71:136–49.
41. Calear AL, Christensen H. Systematic review of school-based prevention and early intervention programs for depression. J Adolesc 2010;33:429–38.
42. Merry S, McDowell H, Hetrick S, et al. Psychological and/or educational interventions for the prevention of depression in children and adolescents. Cochrane Database Syst Rev 2004;1:CD003380.
43. Neil AL, Christensen H. Australian school-based prevention and early intervention programs for anxiety and depression: a systematic review. Med J Aust 2007;186: 305–8.
44. Waddell C, Hua JM, Garland OM, et al. Preventing mental disorders in children: a systematic review to inform policy-making. Can J Public Health 2007;98:166–73.
45. Neil AL, Christensen H. Efficacy and effectiveness of school-based prevention and early intervention programs for anxiety. Clin Psychol Rev 2009;29:208–15.
46. Faggiano F, Vigna-Taglianti FD, Versino E, et al. School-based prevention for illicit drugs' use. Cochrane Database Syst Rev 2005;2:CD003020.
47. Tobler NS, Roona MR, Ochshorn P, et al. School-based adolescent drug prevention programs: 1998 meta-analysis. J Primary Prev 2000;20:275–336.
48. White D, Pitts M. Educating young people about drugs: a systematic review. Addiction 1998;93:1475–87.
49. Mann JJ, Apter A, Bertolote J, et al. Suicide prevention strategies: a systematic review. JAMA 2005;294:2064–74.
50. Robinson J, Hetrick SE, Martin C. Preventing suicide in young people: systematic review. Aust N Z J Psychiatry 2011;45:3–26.
51. Grave RD. School-based prevention programs for eating disorders: achievements and opportunities. Dis Manage Health Outcomes 2003;11:579–93.
52. Pratt BM, Woolfenden SR. Interventions for preventing eating disorders in children and adolescents. Cochrane Database Syst Rev 2002;2:CD002891.

School Law for the Child Psychiatrist: Legal Principles and Case Implications

Colby Brunt, JD[a], Jeffrey Q. Bostic, MD, EdD[b,c],*

KEYWORDS

- School • Mental health • Legal • School law psychiatry
- Special education

As our society becomes more sophisticated, so too do the rules by which we live. Schools struggle with shifting social rules and legal interpretations of what best provides students opportunities while protecting everyone else in the school. Mental health has become a significant topic within schools, because promoting positive mental health, and providing accommodations to those students impacted by an illness—physical or mental—is evolving at an unparalleled pace. Challenges abound around educationally planning for an increasing number of students who have been diagnosed with a psychiatric disorder. Practical issues vary widely among local districts regarding how schools, parents, and clinicians collaborate when a student has, for example, been hospitalized and attempts to return to school, when a student refuses to go to school, or when students require additional supports and services to succeed educationally.

The laws impacting education continue to evolve and to be interpreted differently across the country. At the same time, core tenets and principles appear somewhat consistent across American schools, and clinicians should be familiar with these to best work with schools and to advocate effectively for their patients. This article reviews the current educational law most pertinent to clinicians, and how these principles are applicable in given cases.

FEDERAL LAWS GOVERNING SPECIAL EDUCATION
Individuals with Disabilities Act

In accordance with the federal law regarding special education, the Individuals with Disabilities Education Act (IDEA),[1] a student is found eligible for special education services if a team of individuals (parents, teachers, school staff, and administrators)

[a] Stoneman, Chandler, & Miller LLP
[b] Department of Psychiatry, Harvard Medical School, 6900 Yawkey Building, 55 Fruit Street, Boston, MA 02114, USA
[c] School Psychiatry, Massachusetts General Hospital, Boston, MA, USA
* Corresponding author.
E-mail address: jbostic@partners.org

Child Adolesc Psychiatric Clin N Am 21 (2012) 29–41
doi:10.1016/j.chc.2011.09.001
1056-4993/12/$ – see front matter © 2012 Elsevier Inc. All rights reserved.
childpsych.theclinics.com

find that the student has a disability; is currently not making effective progress in the general education curriculum; and requires special education services to make effective progress in the general education curriculum. Once a student is eligible for special education services, the school district is charged with providing the student a free, appropriate public education (FAPE). Case law defines FAPE as services that provide the student with an educational benefit that enables them to make effective progress toward the general education curriculum.[2] The key issue is that it must enable the student to make effective progress and this may not necessarily be the "best" or most optimal educational program conceivable for the student.

Although eligibility determination seems to be a rather simple set of questions, as with many areas of the law, the legal requirements for schools involving students with mental health issues readily becomes gray. A student may indeed have a disability (such as a serious emotional disturbance [SED]) or the student may not be making progress (perhaps the students has been hospitalized or has been unable to come to school), but the issue that many educational teams face is what special education services the student require to make effective progress. The distinction between educational services and medical services is significant, because clinical needs may require clinical interventions that represent medical services (eg, access to medications when agitated) rather than special education services. For many students, outside medical providers might recommend clinical approaches such as psychiatric interventions or other intensive therapeutic supports. However, case law does not support that a clinical intervention model is something that is necessarily within the purview of schools to provide to students. So the question becomes, where does the school's obligation begin and end for these students?

Under special education law, the range of educational placements and related services vary greatly for students whose primary educational disability is social and/or emotional. For some students, they may require a therapeutic public or private (out-of-district) day placement or a residential placement (24-hour per day school placement) to receive FAPE. First, the educational team must provide an educational plan individualized for a student's needs, and construct an Individualized Educational Program (IEP). Next, the law remains clear that students are to receive the educational services described in the IEP in the "least restrictive setting." Although a residential setting might be the optimal setting for a student, if FAPE can be provided in a day school placement or in a program within the public school, then these less restrictive settings are favored over the more restrictive setting.

In some instances, the team may determine that the student's educational needs are so great that the student can only be served within a residential placement because the student requires 24-hour per day intervention by trained educational staff. Others may require a day placement in a public or private day school that provides the student with a smaller classroom with therapeutic supports throughout the day. Still other students may be able to remain in the public schools with on-site services and supports. For some students, counseling services may be necessary for the student to benefit from his or her educational programming. Usually, such counseling is provided for the student to access the curriculum, rather than to address psychiatric symptoms per se (provide mental health treatment). For example, if a student becomes distraught when math problems become overwhelming, and the student "shuts down" or becomes hostile, that usually falls within the purview of the school; however, if a student reports being persistently suicidal across all settings, that is not recognized as a school issue, but instead a medical issue.[3] Typically, schools have a school adjustment counselor or school psychologist work with the student in a 1:1 setting or within a student group when appropriate. Generally speaking, psychotherapy services that can be performed by counselors or psychologists are considered a "related service" if the service is required in provide the student with a FAPE and to access the curriculum, as opposed to address ongoing mental health needs impacting the child across school, home, and peer domains.

In cases where the family disputes the placement, the student "stays put" in the current placement until resolution occurs. Accordingly, if a family contests the proposed placement (ie, placement within the public school's therapeutic program), the school is not allowed to unilaterally move the student to the proposed placement until the parents agrees to the placement, or until a state due process hearing officer rules in favor of the school or the parent on the appropriate placement. However, parents can choose to place the student elsewhere without going through the team process, to in effect "unilaterally" place the student at their own risk, knowing that the school district may not pay for this placement unless the family can demonstrate that the school's proposed placement was not appropriate and therefore they needed to use "self-help" to place the child themselves. Practically, parents of students who become involved with substance abuse send their child to "boot camps" far away from the student's home. Beyond the risks inherent in unilateral placements, if a distant school is not accredited, or if a closer similar school is accredited in the student's home state, then the school district usually is not required to pay for such unilateral placements. In addition, school districts are typically not required to pay for services and placements that are for the treatment of students with alcohol and substance abuse issues.

IDEA and SED

Under federal law, a student may qualify for special education owing to a finding that the student has an emotional disturbance. An emotional disturbance is defined as a condition exhibiting 1 or more of the following characteristics over a long period of time and to a marked degree that adversely affects a child's educational performance: (1) An inability to learn that cannot be explained by intellectual, sensory, or health factors; (2) an inability to build or maintain satisfactory interpersonal relationships with peers and teachers; (3) inappropriate types of behavior or feelings under normal circumstances; (4) a general pervasive mood of unhappiness or depression; and/or (5) a tendency to develop physical symptoms or fears associated with personal or school problems.[4] It is important for both clinicians and school staff to understand that this is the federal definition under IDEA, and not a diagnosis per the DSM-IV. For many clinicians, it is difficult to understand that schools are governed by the disability definitions outlined in both state and federal education laws. Although a student may carry a diagnosis of depression or anxiety, this may not reach the federal or state definitions of an educational disability, especially if this is not impacting the student while at school; to be found eligible, the student must not be making effective progress in the general education curriculum as a result of the disability. At the same time, these laws do not require a specific diagnosis for a student to be eligible for SED, but instead a "condition" that meets the criteria listed. As a result, a student could have a condition (eg, an emerging paraphilia) that cannot be diagnosed based on age restrictions, yet still qualify for SED. Similarly, students might have more or less severe diagnoses (eg, bipolar disorder), but not be found eligible, whereas a student with dysthymia might instead be categorized SED based on meeting the criteria listed.

Another issue is that neither IDEA nor its regulations define how long a qualifying "long period of time" must be. The Office of Special Education Policy has stated that a generally acceptable definition of "a long period of time" is a range of time from 2 to 9 months, assuming preliminary interventions have been implemented and proven ineffective during that period.[5] This is most frequently modified when a student, not previously eligible for special education services, is hospitalized. Many times, as a part of the student's discharge recommendations, clinicians state that the student requires a residential placement as the next step-down from their hospital level of care. Under the federal disability definition, a hospital stay of even 1 to 2 months does not necessarily qualify the student as SED. In these matters, it is advisable that clinicians engage with school representatives before discharge meetings to discuss appropriate next steps for the student, including a discussion about educational services and/or a referral to special education for an sevaluation.

Case example 1
A high school junior who has never been found eligible for special education services was hospitalized for 2 weeks and then released to a step-down program. While in the step-down program, her parents reached out to the school to secure a residential placement per the recommendation of the treatment team at the step-down facility. The school held an emergency team meeting, and agreed to find the student eligible and placed her on a partial IEP with an extended initial evaluation at a residential facility. The school and parents agreed that they needed additional information as to the student's condition and educational needs and where she could receive her education and services in the least restrictive environment. The school proposed the evaluation to take place over 8 weeks. During her evaluation period, the student stabilized and she was successful during the school day at the residential facility. As a result, the school-based team, the parents, and the clinicians were able to facilitate a step-down transition for the student to return home and attend a therapeutic day placement.

STUDENT DISCIPLINE AND SPECIAL EDUCATION

With respect to issues involving student discipline, there are additional protections for the following students: (1) Students who are eligible for special education, (2) students who the school might have had prior knowledge that they might be eligible for special education, and (3) those that are in the referral/evaluation process for special education. If a student described in 1 to 3 above violates the code of conduct and the student is going to suspended for longer than 10 schools days or has accumulated more than 10 school days of suspension for incidents that were close in time and similar in offense, the school must convene a team to conduct a "manifestation determination." The team must determine whether (1) the conduct was a direct result of the school's failure to implement the IEP or (2) the conduct was caused by, or had a direct and substantial relationship to, the student's disability. Simply put, if the answer is yes to either question, then the school cannot remove that student from his or her current placement for longer than 10 days, unless the student brought a weapon or illegal drugs to school or caused serious bodily injury to another while at school. In these circumstances, the principal can remove the student for 45 school days to an interim alternative setting. Similarly, if there is an issue of danger (danger to self or others), then the school can proceed to an expedited due process hearing to seek a change in placement. If the conduct in question is not a manifestation of the disability (eg, a student with a reading disability gets into a serious fight), or if it is not a direct result of the school's failure to implement the IEP (eg, the school failed to provide reading services and the student got into a fight in the lunchroom), then the school can suspend the student as they would any other student; however, the school is still obligated to provide FAPE (eg, tutoring, alternative placement).

SECTION 504 OF THE REHABILITATION ACT OF 1973

Section 504 of The Rehabilitation Act of 1973 mandates that schools cannot deny a student access to a program or service solely on the basis of the student's disability. Unlike IDEA, Section 504 provides students with accommodations to allow them access to the average program or service; that is, under Section 504 a student may receive accommodations to help that student do what other students do (eg, extended time to do the same test), versus changes in the curricular requirements (ie, modifications) available for students under IDEA, who may not be able to reach the same expectations of other students. Commonly, students with disabilities such as attention deficit hyperactivity disorder may be provided a 504 plan and receive accommodations (to achieve the same expectations academically of other students), such as increased time, seating at the front of the class, a box with supplies in the classroom, and a separate set of books/materials at home to address their disability. For "episodic" issues, such as students with separation anxiety that emerges at the beginning of each school year, a 504 plan may better fit the needs of these students. A 504 plan is not inferior to an IEP or a "consolation prize" should the student not be eligible for special education, but rather a more appropriate option for students who require accommodations to access the general education curriculum and who do not require specialized instruction. Distinctions between IDEA and 504 plans are summarized in **Table 1**.

RESPONSE TO INTERVENTION

Response to Intervention (RTI) is a model process that allows for early detection and response to students' learning and behavioral difficulties within the general education classroom by providing high-quality instruction in suspected areas of need and gathering data to monitor the effectiveness of the interventions.[6] Schools use RTI to quickly determine whether a student may be eligible for special education or whether short-term, focused interventions may be enough to help the student to "catch up" if the student is not keeping pace academically. The core concepts of RTI are: (1) Application of scientific, research based interventions in the general education classroom; (2) measurement of a student's response to these interventions; and (3) use of the RTI data to inform instruction.[7] RTI incorporates a 3-tier model. Tier 1 includes high-quality instruction and behavioral supports in the general education classroom (ie, best teaching practices). Tier 2 includes more specialized instruction for students whose performance and rate of progress is lagging compared to their peers (eg, remedial reading instruction; counseling). Tier 3 includes comprehensive evaluation by a multidisciplinary team to determine whether the student has a disability and is eligible for special education and related services. The benefit to RTI is that it helps with the early identification of, and rapid response to, students who may require special education services; typically, RTI assists in the reduction in the number of special education students, and the use of RTI in the classroom and the data gathered from these interventions provides instructionally relevant information for all students with respect to their educational planning. Specifically for students with emotional needs, RTI interventions may include counseling services, social pragmatic groups, a short-term general education therapeutic program, or even a modified (shorter) day.

Table 1
Educational distinctions between IDEA and section 504

	IDEA	Section 504
What is the purpose of the law?	To provide an eligible student was specialized instruction or services in order to make effective progress toward the general education curriculum.	To provide an eligible student with necessary accommodations to allow the student access to the general education curriculum or program.
Who is an eligible student?	(i) Student with a disability per state and federal special education regulations, (ii) who is not making progress in the general education curriculum as a result of the disability, and (iii) needs specialized instruction or related services to make progress.	(i) Student with an impairment or is regarded as having an impairment, (ii) that substantially limits ≥1 major life activities (learning, reading, concentrating, etc); and (iii) requires accommodations in order to access the programs and services as the average nondisabled peers.
What defines if student has a disability or impairment?	Teams are bound by the disability definitions per state and federal special education regulations.	An impairment is a medical/educational/ psychological/ psychiatric diagnosis (ie, may rely on DSM-IV diagnosis).
What evaluations are needed to determine eligibility?	An educational assessment and assessments in all suspected areas of need. Must have consent from parents to conduct testing.	District must use valid, relevant tests and other evaluation information. Schools cannot rely solely on a note from a doctor. Must have consent from parents to conduct testing.
Who is on the school-based "team"?	Must invite: Parents, special education teacher, regular education (if student is included with non-disabled peers or may be included with nondisabled peers); may invite, when appropriate evaluators (in school and private); eligible student (typically >14 years old); specialists in school (counselors, speech-language pathologists, etc), and any other individual with knowledge of child at parent or school request.	Persons knowledgeable about the student, evaluation data and/or service/accommodation options.

What is FAPE?	A program designed to provide and educational benefit.	A program as adequate as provided for average, nondisabled peers.
Does the plan itself require parent/guardian consent?	Yes.	No. Under the law there is no requirement that a 504 plan be in writing. However, it is best practice for schools to put it in writing.
When must the school implement the plan?	Once the school has received parental consent, the plan must be implemented immediately.	The school must implement the plan immediately.
What if the parent disagrees with the plan?	Parent can accept in full, reject in full, or reject in part. Whatever has been accepted must be implemented immediately. If the plan is rejected the student is entitled to "stay put" in last agreed upon placement and/or services until resolved between the parties or through a due process hearing at the state.	Parent can file for a due process hearing with the state regarding their disagreement. There is no "stay put" right under 504; therefore, the school implements the plan as proposed until the parties agree or a hearing officer states otherwise.

SPECIFIC EXAMPLES OF SCHOOL-RELATED PSYCHIATRIC CASES
School Phobia/Avoidance Cases

Schools, parents, and clinicians often struggle to manage school phobia or school avoidant cases. Schools rely on clinicians to discern whether the student is not attending school because of a phobia versus truancy; students with anxiety and who fear separation from a parent or fear humiliation in class (classic anxiety) are managed differently from students who avoid attending school because they prefer to spend time with their peers outside school (eg, gang activities) during school hours (classic truancy). School refusal or school phobia typically involves emotional distress about attending; the parents are aware that the student is not attending school, the student is not showing significant antisocial behaviors, the child remains at home during the school day, and the child expresses a desire and willingness to complete work. Unlike school refusal cases, in truancy cases the student does not have anxiety regarding attending school; these children typically attempt to conceal that they are not attending school from the parent, the child does not usually remain at home during the school day (although they may sleep in during school hours), and the child typically demonstrates a lack of interest in his or her education.[8] Accordingly, clinicians must first discern whether the student is not going to school or cannot go to school. Once the clinician has clarified "why" the student is not attending, then focus on the "how" of getting the student back into school can be addressed with school staff. With respect to the "how," clinicians are most helpful to schools when they review medical, educational (including attendance reports, report cards, any special education records or evaluations, and correspondence between the family and school), and any legal documents (eg, truancy filings, criminal records, divorce/family court records), and speak with the student, parents, other providers, and school staff. Although this can be time-consuming, clinicians who integrate relevant medical, educational, and legal materials, are most credible to schools and best able to have their recommendations implemented. Although clinicians often have recommendations that are likely to be helpful, schools are not mandated to follow the recommendations of a clinician, but instead to rely on the wider educational team to decide and implement recommendations.

From the school's perspective, legal mandates require schools to ensure that children who are school age (typically 6–16 years old) attend school on a regular basis, and for those who are eligible for special education be provided with FAPE in accordance with state and federal special education laws. For example, if the student who is of mandatory school age and has been absent for a certain number of school days (typically 7–14) without an identified reason (eg, medical illness such as pneumonia), the school district is required to file notice of this "truancy" with the juvenile court. Once that occurs, the student and the family must answer to the court why the student has been absent and, in many instances, make an agreement with the court and probation for the student to attend school on a regular basis.

Students may need to remain at home for a medical reason (eg, during chemotherapy treatments or when a student remains contagious to others [school refusal is ordinarily not perceived a contagious disease]). However, clinicians should avoid writing excuses for a child to remain at home if it is not medically necessary. For example, in some states, if a student is going to be out of school for longer than 14 school days, the parent may submit a "home–hospital" form to obtain home tutoring from the school. Home–hospital forms are completed by a doctor who states that a student is either confined to the home or hospital for medical reasons for a period of 14 days or longer or for intermittent periods of time throughout the school year.[9]

Although the intent of the home–hospital forms have been to provide tutoring to children who are out of school for a medical reason, schools increasingly contest the validity of these forms when they seem to be used to perpetuate the student's continued absence from school. The following case illuminates the recent findings of courts around these issues.[10]

Case example 2

A high school student diagnosed with a mood disorder and pervasive developmental disorder NOS was on an individualized education plan since first grade, and was most recently placed in the high school substantially separate therapeutic program. Within his program, he receives counseling, a social skills group, and is heavily supported in co-taught "inclusion" (regular education with special educators co-teaching with the regular teacher) classes. In addition to his school program, the school also provides in-home parent training to assist the parent with the student at home. The home program focuses on a behavioral plan that can be implemented at home and at school. After the student was hospitalized for 1 week for behavioral issues in the home, his doctor submitted a home–hospital tutoring form to the school stating the student could not return to school "until the school found an appropriate placement." The parent admitted she was overwhelmed and wanted a residential placement, although the school district continued to propose its therapeutic placement as least restrictive to keep the student within the community. The student remained out of school for 4 months while the parties disputed the appropriate placement. The hearing officer found that the school's proposed placement was appropriate because the parent was unable to prove that the student required a residential placement for educational purposes. The hearing officer also ruled that the home–hospital forms the parent submitted were invalid because there was no medical reason the student was confined to the home and that simply stating that the placement was not appropriate was not a legally valid reason to require the school to provide home tutoring.

In addition to cases involving students who are out of school through a doctor's order (eg, home–hospital form), there are cases where all parties agree that the student needs to be in school, but for some reason the student is unable to physically enter the school or remain in school (eg, school phobia/avoidance). The key issue in these cases is that parents, clinicians, and school staff immediately address the issue before the student completely stopping school attendance. If the school starts to see a pattern of absences, schools need to immediately convene a meeting with school staff, parents, and outside providers/clinicians to try to discern why the student is not coming to school. Based on this meeting, the school may then want to propose an evaluation, such as a psychological evaluation or a functional behavioral assessment, to determine why the student is not coming to school from an educational perspective and what the adults (school staff, clinicians, parents) can do to assist the student with transitioning back into an education program. These evaluations need to focus on the "why" (eg, Is the student being bullied by another student? Is the student experiencing debilitating anxiety owing to academic pressure? ?does the student have an aversion to a large building/classroom? Is there some recent trauma that the student has experienced?) and the "how" (eg, Does the student need a reduced day to transfer back in, or a different placement, and/or require counseling in school?), and to further consider the "function" of the behavior (ie, what the student "gains" by remaining at home and what makes that preferable to going to school). Sometimes students are avoiding school because of variables there, but also they may prefer something at home (playing video games instead of doing school work) or in the community (hanging out with peers) to going to school. Ultimately, all parties need to work together to assist the student with transitioning back into an educational placement as soon as the student is able; the longer students are out of an educational placement, the harder it is for them transition back and be successful.[11]

Case example 3
A fifth-grade student stopped coming to school. The school reached out to the parents after the student had been absent for 24 school days (all excused by various doctors' notes). The parents informed the school that the student did not feel safe being away from her parents because she feared her parent might "die." The parents informed the school that the student's aunt had passed away suddenly the previous summer, this had a profoundly effected the student, and the student began weekly outside counseling. The school sought a release to speak to the student's therapist and requested that the district's consulting psychiatrist speak to the therapist to assist the school with educational planning for the student. The student's therapist recommended that the student return to school with the assistance of a desensitization plan involving at least 1 parent's presence in school throughout the day. Although highly unusual to have a parent in school throughout the school day, the school agreed to move forward with the plan. The therapist and school district's staff worked collaboratively to develop a plan and, more important, that family and the school could both support when presenting it to the student.

Aligning the family, student, and the school to facilitate reentry to the school as soon as possible optimizes successful and quicker returns in school refusal cases. The sooner that the student reenters a school environment, with the support and cohesive efforts of school, parents, and providers, the greater the probability that the student will continue in school and be successful.

CONDUCT DISORDER/SOCIAL MALADJUSTMENT CASES

A particularly problematic area for schools and providers involves cases where students seem to be socially maladjusted as evidenced by disordered behavior. The case law in this area tends to find students ineligible for special education services when their behaviors seem to be primarily the result of what is characterized as disruptive disordered behavior. IDEA specifically states that disability category of "SED" does not apply to children who are socially maladjusted.[12] However, where clinicians and educators may disagree is that clinicians may term the student's disability, under the DSM-IV, as conduct disorder or oppositional defiant disorder, and thus disagreement ensues as to whether the student has an educationally defined disability verses a DSM-IV disability. Again, schools are held to the disability definitions within state and federal regulations; in many instances, these students are not eligible for special education services. As the Federal Office of Special Education Programs (Office of Special Education Policy) stated in response to this issue and how it relates to eligibility: "[T]he essential element appears to be the student's inability to control his/her behavior (*Doe v. Maher,* 793 F.2d 1470, 1480 footnote 8, (9th Cir. 1986)) and conform his/her conduct to socially acceptable norms (*Honig v. Doe,* 108 S.Ct. 592, 595 (1988)). However, a student exhibiting such behaviors is eligible for special education and related services only if they meet the additional criteria contained in the [SED] definition (34 CFR §§ 300.5(b)(8))."[13]

Although students who exhibit socially maladjusted behavior may not be eligible under IDEA, there is guidance from the Federal Department of Education Office of Civil Rights that support that a student may be eligible under Section 504 of the Rehabilitation Act of 1973.[14] In the matter of Irvine (CA) Unified Sch. Dist., the Office of Civil Rights found that a student with social maladjustment could be covered under

Section 504 if the student has been diagnosed as having a disorder, because under Section 504 the student need only to establish that his or her social maladjustment was a mental impairment, which substantially limited a major life activity, such as his ability to learn or attend school.[15]

Case example 4

A high school senior who was previously eligible for a 504 Plan owing to attention deficit hyperactivity disorder during middle school, was found ineligible under 504 in his freshman year. The student was arrested on school grounds for possession of marijuana with the intent to distribute marijuana. Under the code of conduct in the student handbook and state law, the principal of the high school moved to expel the student from school. Before his expulsion hearing, the attorney for the student and the parents requested a special education evaluation, which the district then provided. The education team found that the student was within the average range on all academic testing and the psychological assessment found that the student was in the average range cognitively. However, the rating scales in the psychological evaluation that were completed by the parents and teachers indicated that the student was in the clinically significant range for conduct problems and school problems. The team also reviewed the students grades (mostly Ds and Fs) and attendance (student was absent 5 school days, tardy 15 times, and dismissed 3). The student admitted that he was using marijuana on a daily basis. Although the student was not getting good grades and was using drugs, the school-based team determined that he was not eligible because he did not have a disability under state and federal definitions. The parents disagreed with the finding and sent the student to a residential placement focusing on drug and alcohol rehabilitation. The parents requested that the school pay for the placement and sought a hearing that to determine this issue.

The hearing officer found that the student was not eligible under IDEA because the student did not have a disability in accordance with state and federal laws. The hearing officer declined to order the school district to reimburse the parents for the cost of the residential placement, but ordered the school district to convene a 504 Team to determine whether the student would be eligible under Section 504 for an accommodation plan. The hearing officer declined to rule on the issue of whether a drug and alcohol rehabilitation facility would be appropriate for educational reasons.

COMMUNICATION AND THE HEALTH INSURANCE PORTABILITY AND ACCOUNTABILITY ACT

Communication among providers, school personnel, and families is key to assisting students through their school careers. A recent American Academy of Child and Adolescent Psychiatry Practice Parameter[16] regarding the use of psychotropic medication in children and adolescents has listed communication with other professionals, including educators, as a key principle for clinicians to employ. It is paramount that the clinicians work with parents to ensure that the necessary releases are secured for this communication. As clinicians are aware, they are bound by the Health Insurance Portability and Accountability Act,[17] whereas schools for the most part are not, but rather are bound by state and federal laws and regulations regarding student records. The federal student records law, the Family Education Rights Privacy Act,[18] denies most third-party access to student records without the consent of the parent. Without a valid release, both clinicians' and schools' hands are tied; as such, the communication lines are severed. Schools and clinicians should work with the parents to obtain releases, even if the releases are limited (eg, a release that only allows the clinician to speak with specific school staff, such as a school psychologist or school physician), so that the parent feels that they are not signing over the student's entire medical history to the school, yet the school is able to get the information necessary for educational planning.

RECOMMENDING INTERVENTIONS AND SCHOOL PROGRAMS

It is important for clinicians to be aware of what educational programs are available for students within, as well as beyond, a school district. Unfortunately, without communication between clinicians and the schools, clinicians may rely solely on the parents or the student regarding what the student's current educational programming is or what the school has to offer. School personnel are usually much more familiar with the continuum of services available within the public school district, and districts often establish relationships with "out-of-district" placements where they send multiple students and can have more consistent and frequent communication. Among the most frustrating complaints levied toward clinicians by school staff is when a clinician recommends a specific out-of-school placement for a patient, and without speaking to anyone at the student's school. What is much more helpful is for clinicians to describe the interventions that a student requires, rather than to name a school placement. Clinicians should recommend particular services or supports that the student may require, rather than just recommending a specific school. This approach can be very helpful in advocating for the student's needs and for the district to identify appropriate placements.

TRANSITIONAL PROGRAMS

Many schools now are working with clinicians to develop programs to educate students with emotional disorders. For example, some schools have programs that are specifically developed for students to reenter school after a hospitalization. Typically, these programs have school adjustment counselors or school psychologists on site available to the students throughout the day. This helps students to transition slowly into regular education classes as appropriate, and if necessary, to allow students to spend time within a small classroom or classrooms to complete class work when the student cannot tolerate being in a larger, regular education classroom. For many students, this temporary program allows the student to transition at a pace that can be titrated as the regular school stressors emerge yet with the support of school clinicians.

DISTRICT THERAPEUTIC PROGRAMS

Increasingly, school districts are developing in-district therapeutic programs. These programs typically provide what many refer to as a "home-base" approach, meaning that the students in the program can access a "therapeutic homeroom" throughout the day as needed. Most in-district therapeutic programs provide small group academic classes, resource room support when students have difficult days, group and individual counseling sessions throughout the school week, and classes specifically geared to addressing the students' social and emotional needs within academic courses. For some students, they may only require accessing some counseling services and resource room support, whereas others may require having all classes within the program. The benefit to an in-district therapeutic program is that it allows the students to remain in their communities and provides flexibility for students to both increase their time in the inclusion setting (ie, general education classes) as needed, as well as access additional services within the therapeutic program if necessary without needing to be removed to a more restrictive day placement (that limits the student's involvement in extracurricular activities, with local peers, and the community). As with all students, the goal is for students to be educated within the general education setting to the greatest extent possible in preparation for participation in "regular life."

SUMMARY

Regardless of special education designations for students, clinicians are most helpful to their patients when they effectively partner with the individual student, family, and school team members to provide the youth with the supports necessary to make effective educational progress. By coalescing the educational team, the clinician optimizes the range of options available for each student. Students' needs change as they proceed through different developmental stages, so the ongoing school–clinician–family relationship provides the widest array of school experiences for students, and gives the opportunity for school programs to evolve in addressing the emerging needs of students. Familiarity with the parameters for finding students eligible for special educational services, and for managing returns from hospitalization, home-based services, and diverse in- and out-of-district options, helps to position the clinician to best partner with families and school staff and advocate most effectively for their patients.

REFERENCES

1. 20 USC 1400 et. seq.; 34 CFR 300 et. Seq.
2. Board of Education v. Rowley, 458 US 176 (1982).
3. See 34 CFR 300.34(c)(10); Max M. v. Thompson, 556 IDELR 227 (N.D. Ill. 1984); TG v. Board of Educ., 555 IDELR 391 (D.N.J. 1983); and Papacoda v. Connecticut, 552 IDELR 495 (D. Conn. 1981).
4. 34 CFR 300.8 (c)(4)(i).
5. Letter to Anonymous, 213 IDELR 247 (Office of Special Education Policy 1989).
6. Questions and Answers on Response to Intervention and Early Intervening Services (EIS), 47 IDELR 196 (OSER 2007).
7. National Joint Committee on Leaning Disabilities. Responsiveness to intervention and learning disabilities. Washington (DC): National Joint Committee on Leaning Disabilities; 2005.
8. Fremont WP. School refusal in children and adolescents. Am Fam Physician 2003; 68:1555–61.
9. 603 CMR 28.03(3)(c).
10. 15 MSER 259, 267 (MA SEA, 2009, Figueroa).
11. Fremont, citing Kennedy WA. School phobia: rapid treatment of fifty cases. J Abnorm Psychol 1965;70:285–9.
12. 34 CFR 300.8(c)(4)(ii).
13. Letter to Anonymous, 213 IDELR 247 (Office of Special Education Policy, 1989).
14. 29 U. S.C. § 794.
15. 353 IDELR 192 (Office of Civil Rights, 1989).
16. American Academy of Child and Adolescent Psychiatry. Practice parameter on the use of psychotropic medication in children and adolescents. J Am Acad Child Adolesc Psychiatry 2009;48:961–73.
17. PL 104-191.
18. 20 U. S.C. § 1232g.

Spinning Our Wheels: Improving Our Ability to Respond to Bullying and Cyberbullying

Elizabeth K. Englander, PhD

KEYWORDS

• Abuse • Bullying • Cyberbullying • School response

Bullying and aggression in schools today has reached epidemic proportions.[1] Although always in existence, bullying behaviors have increased in frequency and in severity in the past few decades.[2] Abusive bullying behaviors begin in elementary school, peak during middle school, and begin to subside as children progress through their high school years.[3] Nationwide statistics suggest that somewhere between 1 in 6 and 1 in 4 students are frequently bullied at school.[1] The 2005 Youth Risk Behavior Survey in Massachusetts found that 24% of teenagers reported being bullied at schools in the year before the survey. A study of 21,000 Massachusetts schoolchildren between October 2010 and February 2011 found that about one fourth of middle- and high-schoolers reported being physically bullied, and more than double that number reported being taunted or called a name (**Fig. 1**).[4]

The problem does not seem to be improving. In that a 2007 survey, 54% of Massachusetts schools indicated that bullying has become more of a problem "in the last few years."[5] Another study found that most children who were bullied were victimized for 6 months or longer (Mullin-Rindler N. Findings from the Massachusetts Bullying Prevention Initiative. Unpublished manuscript; 2003). The US Department of Education has found that bullying increased 5% between 1999 and 2001[6] and the National Education Association has suggested that bullying is a serious problem in US schools.[7]

Bullying behaviors are associated with catastrophic violence. In the 2004–2005 school year, 24 school deaths in the United States were the result of shootings,[8] and the most common reason students bring weapons to school is protection against bullies.[9] We now know that the school shooters of the 1990s often reported being the chronic victims of bullies.[3] In the 1990s, a string of copycat shootings in suburban and

Massachusetts Aggression Reduction Center, Bridgewater State University, Bridgewater, MA 02325, USA
E-mail address: MARC@bridgew.edu

Child Adolesc Psychiatric Clin N Am 21 (2012) 43–55
doi:10.1016/j.chc.2011.08.013
1056-4993/12/$ – see front matter
childpsych.theclinics.com

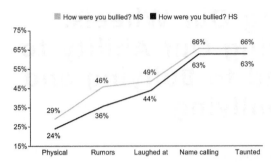

Fig. 1. How were you bullied?

rural school districts caused enormous alarm and dismay and, although more recent attacks have been averted, vigilance and fear remain high.[10]

WHAT IS BULLYING?

Bullying is the physical and or psychological abuse, perpetuated by 1 powerful child upon another, with the intention to harm or dominate. Typically, bullying is repetitive, intentional, and involves an imbalance of power.[11] Bullies enjoy social power and therefore seek out situations where they can dominate others. Bullying can be either direct, such as physical or verbal aggression, or indirect, such as insults, threats, name calling, spreading rumors, or encouraging exclusion from a peer group.[2]

It is unfortunate that adults often consider bullying an inevitable and even normal part of childhood. This belief undoubtedly stems from memories of the qualitative bullying of past generations, which was much less frequent, less supported by children's peers, conducted by socially ostracized children, and never, of course, online. Little wonder that adults today frequently ask why "such a fuss" is made over bullying—which is, as they recall it, an unpleasant but infrequent childhood behavior. One result of this attitude is that adults sometimes fail to intervene—resulting in the victim feeling powerless and hopeless in a situation that is torturous in nature.[12] If children feel powerless in situations that adults perceive yet dismiss, how much more powerless must they feel when they are victimized in a way that adults cannot even begin to comprehend?

Bullying Today is Different from Bullying in Previous Generations

Bullies today are popular and socially successful in a way that they have not been in past generations.[13] The popularity of bullies is without a doubt a significant change, but it pales in comparison to the significance of the dawn of the age of cyber immersion. *Cyber immersion* refers to the utilization of cyber technology and the Internet as a central, rather than as an adjunct, element of daily life.[14] The generational shift from cyber *utilization* (using the Internet as a convenience and an adjunct to real life) to cyber *immersion* (using the Internet as a primary or central method of communication, commerce, relationships, and recreation) is a generational shift that has not seen its equal since the Sexual Revolution in the 1960s and 1970s or the turn-of-the-century immigration into the United States. Then, as now, the older generation lacks a basic understanding of how the younger generation is thinking, feeling, and acting. This ignorance adds an additional layer of obstacles to the work that adults must do to combat childhood abusiveness or bullying.

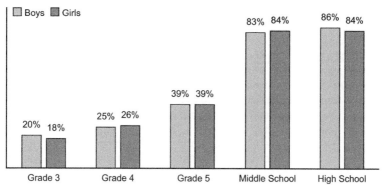

Fig. 2. Access to computers and mobile devices begins early.

What Do We Need to Know About Cyberbullying and Online Behaviors between Children?

Cyberbullying has emerged as 1 result of the increasingly online social life in which modern teens and children engage. Teens reported having received threatening messages, having had private e-mails or messages forwarded without their consent; having had an embarrassing picture of themselves posted online without their consent; or having had rumors spread about them online.[15] Because online teenage life is ever-present among First-World teenagers, cyberbullying may become—or may even already be—the dominant form of bullying behavior among children. Access to computers and mobile devices begins young; about 19% of third graders "own" cell phones (**Fig. 2**) and more than 90% of third graders play online games in a study in Massachusetts.[4]

Is cyberbullying more common than schoolyard bullying? A recent telephone study of 886 US Internet users age 12 to 17 (conducted October to November 2006) found that one third (32%) of all teenagers who use the Internet say they have been targeted for cyberbullying online.[15] Another 2006 survey of 18- and 19-year-old college freshman found that 40% reported having been "harassed, bullied, stalked, or threatened via instant messaging."[16] One fifth (20%) of the respondents in that study also admitted being a cyberbully themselves. Over two thirds (73%) had seen an insulting, threatening, or degrading profile on a social networking website such as MySpace. A follow-up MARC survey in 2007 of undergraduate students found that 24% admitted to cyberbullying and that, again, 40% admitted to being victimized online. A 2006 poll of 1000 children conducted by *Fight Crime: Invest in Kids*, found cyberbullying frequencies of about 33%, similar to those found by Pew and MARC.[15] These numbers suggest that cyberbullying (with about 35%–40% admitting victimization) may be more common than traditional bullying (with about 20%–24% admitting victimization).

In another survey,[5] most cyberbullying perpetrators attributed their online bullying to either anger (65%) or "a joke" (35%) with "revenge" and "no reason" being distant third choices. More than two thirds of students knew a friend who had been victimized online and almost one fourth (24%) characterized cyberbullying as either prevalent or very prevalent in their high school. Even if cyberbullying is more prevalent than in-person bullying, the focus of cyberbullying seems to be similar to the focus of bullying: The most common foci for cyberbullies were someone's appearance and/or who they dated or befriended.

Cyberbullying seems to evoke bullying behaviors among some adolescents who otherwise might not bully. Only 13% of the college students in MARC's 2007 study (above) expressed the opinion that most cyberbullies "would bully no matter what"; instead, they saw bullying online as an opportunistic crime ("easier because you do not see the person" [69%], or done because "you can do it anonymously" [65%]). More than two thirds of the respondents (72%) characterized cyberbullies as predominantly female—a stark contrast to the traditional view that males predominant in aggression.[16] Females seem to use cyberbullying predominately for revenge, whereas boys used it mostly "as a joke." These data suggest that different approaches may need to be tried with boys and girls regarding cyberbullying, and that it "attracts" more female offenders than traditional bullying ever did. Clearly, cyberbullying throws a wider net than traditional "in-person" aggression, and more and different types of offenders should be expected to emerge.

How Do We Measure Who is a Bully and Who is Not?

Many theoreticians have offered typologies of bullies (**Fig. 3**). The following typology has been utilized[17] in response to the advent of cyberbullying and the resulting comparisons that now occur between schoolyard (traditional) bullying and cyberbullying. Traditional psychological theory might hold that the vehicle is of less importance than the intent; that is, if one wants to be a bully, then one finds a vehicle (schoolyard or cyber)—and if a vehicle is unavailable another will be used (eg, if one cannot bully

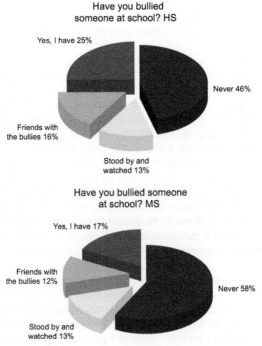

Fig. 3. Types of bullying behavior.

online then one bullies in person). The motivation is paramount. Other psychological theories emphasize the opportunistic situation more (ie, that some types of bullying only occur when the situation permits or encourages them), and these theories seem to "fit" better with cyberbullying, because many cyberbullies do not choose in-person bullying if the cyber route is denied.[16]

It is notable that some experts have already identified patterns of differences between children who only bully online and children who bully in person or both in person and online.[18] In working with schools, MARC finds it useful to identify 5 types of bullies.

Bullies
These children are "traditional" schoolyard bullies. Their motivation is to dominate over their victims, increase their own social status, and instill fear in potential victims. Their modus operandi is to abuse their victims, either physically or (more commonly) psychologically/verbally. As a group, they tend to have high self-esteem and a marked tendency to perceive themselves as under attack in a hostile environment.[19] Their academic achievement may be moderate to poor, and aggression is their preferred tool for domination. They rely on peer support or lack of intervention to continue their activities. Limit-setting is the adult response which operates best to reduce this type of bullying behavior.[2]

Eggers
"Eggers" (referred to by Olweus as "henchmen" or "followers") are so called because their main function is to egg on bullies. These children are a primary support system for schoolyard bullies. Eggers often have poor self-esteem and poor social skills. They befriend and assist bullies because they fear being victimized and because by doing so they gain a high-status, socially powerful friend. Unlike bullies, they do not see their own bullying behaviors as a justified response to a hostile world; they accurately perceive that their behaviors are harmful and unacceptable, but they tend to minimize their own involvement or minimize the impact of their own behaviors. Although some eggers are consistently friendly with a bully, a subtype are floaters. Floaters are not regular friends of bullies, but who may egg on or help bullies during specific bullying situations because they fear being victimized themselves, or because they see it as socially desirable to help out popular bullies. They may "float" in and out of helping bullies; in some situations, they may be a silent bystander, whereas in others, they may actively assist the bully (eg, by laughing at a victim). Like all eggers, they minimize the damage their behavior causes and try to avoid self-confrontation regarding their own role in bullying. Floaters may be "unintentional cyberbullies" as well (see below).

All-around bullies
All-around bullies are schoolyard bullies who are widening their bullying activities into the electronic realm (ie, cyberbullying). Their motivation and modus operandi are the same as bullies; they simply regard the electronic realm as a new arena of opportunity to continue their abusive activities.

Only-cyberbullies
Only-cyberbullies are children who would not engage in schoolyard bullying, but do engage in cyberbullying because they have a set of beliefs or attitudes that support cyberbullying specifically. For example, only-cyberbullies might not bully in person because they are powerless socially or invested in school and academics, yet they are willing to bully online because they believe that cyberbullying is without risk, because

adults are seen as simply not being part of the virtual world. The only-cyberbully could be a victim of an in-person bully at school, who attacks his tormenter online, where he can do so relatively safely.

Unintentional cyberbullies

These children also cyberbully because of a set of beliefs or attitudes, but they seem to do so without the intent to actively bully that characterizes only-cyberbullies. One common attitude in this group is that the Internet "does not count" or "is not real" and so what happens there does not particularly hurt anybody or carry any risks. Because of their limited ability to apply their own victimization experiences, children may believe these myths even when they themselves have been hurt online. Alternatively, some unintentional cyberbullies may truly be intending to joke but their writing does not convey their tone accurately, and their words are taken seriously even though they were not always intended to be taken that way. We know that many adults are overconfident that their writing accurately reflects its intended emotional tone,[20] and it is reasonable to assume that children make similarly poor judgments.

How Might Some of Our Current Responses be Exacerbating the Problems of Bullying and Cyberbullying?

Educators in the United States today are encouraged to utilize mediation techniques in addressing student conflicts, particularly at the high school and middle school levels. Some teachers are incorporating conflict resolution and mediation and negotiation techniques into standard curriculum.[21] Research has generally found a high level of satisfaction with Peer Mediation programs in school-based settings.[22] Programs that include teacher training have often emphasized the role that teachers can take in using medication and negotiation between children who are in conflict.[23] There has been a definitive trend toward training students and teachers to use mediation as the best method to resolve conflict in schools.[24]

The very real success of this trend, in general, discourages critical evaluation of the effectiveness of mediation and negotiation in different types of conflicts among students. However, researchers have discovered that several factors significantly inhibit the use of mediation in schools.[25] One such factor seems to be conflicts that involve bullying.

Mediation and negotiation generally assume that the 2 children in conflict possess relatively equal power, but bullying episodes are defined by their imbalance of power.[11] Theberge and Karan[25(p5)] note that "power imbalances inhibit the use of mediation." This power imbalance renders mediation and negotiation often inappropriate for both the bully and the target.

Many experts in this field have asserted that mediation is not the ideal approach to resolve a bullying situation[26] because a bully may be adept at being charming or lying during a mediation.[27] Rather than being candid and upfront, bullies may work hard outside of the mediation to attain their goal of dominance over the target.[27]

From the victim's point of view, their fear of retribution may make it impossible for them to participate fully, because mediation and negotiation require both parties to assert their own needs and to be frank about their problems with the other party's behavior. A useful analogy is the case of spousal abuse. Would we require a victim of domestic violence to report openly on a violent individual while still living with him or her? There is a general understanding that a victim who refuses to testify is behaving out of fear of retribution, not out of indifference to her condition. Similarly, requiring targets of bullies to "rat out" a bully in a mediation session while continuing to "live" with the bully on a daily basis in the same school is probably an unreasonable request. Part of the teacher training in the Massachusetts Aggression Reduction Center (MARC) (Elizabeth K. Englander. Coping with aggression and bullying as a teacher [personal communication, Massachusetts Aggression Reduction Center, Bridgewater State College, Bridgewater, MA, 2004]). involves raising awareness about why victims of bullies may dismiss, minimally participate, or refuse to participate in mediation; they are not indifferent to their situation, but rather, targets may resist negotiations because they fear retribution and revenge too vividly.

Mediation and negotiation also do not help the child with stable aggressive tendencies—that is, such an approach does not help a bully, but rather, may compound their problems. Children who are stably aggressive have a marked tendency to regard themselves as either victims or as responding appropriately to nakedly hostile threats.[28] This "aggressor-as-victim" style is the direct result of a cognitive tendency to misinterpret ambiguous events as hostile attacks.[28,29] Thus, rather than suffering from poor self-esteem, bullies tend to regard themselves as reacting appropriately.[30] They see mediation and negotiation as appeasement and tend not to take it seriously (Elizabeth K. Englander. Coping with aggression and bullying as a teacher [personal communication, Massachusetts Aggression Reduction Center, Bridgewater State College, Bridgewater, MA, 2004]). The corrective goal should be, therefore, not to validate the bully's perceptions but rather to challenge the validity of their responses. Jane Bluestein's work[31] on "emotional intelligence" suggests that bullies may use emotional information to facilitate their hypersensitivity to hostile cues in the environment, but that such tendencies can be "untaught."

In summary, mediation may be inappropriate for a few reasons. First, it relies on candor and a willingness to acknowledge the other party's point of view—something generally lacking in bullies (but not always; see below). Also, it often seeks to emphasize to each party the validity of the other point of view, when work on biased misperceptions and emotional intelligence suggests that bullies need to understand the biases inherent in their own points of view, rather than to have them validated. Although many educators have long approached conflict in children through the use of mediation and negotiation, discipline through limit setting may be the only effective means of encouraging children to cease bullying others. Although aggressive children may (in part) behave that way because of past exposure to inconsistent discipline, research suggests that firm limit setting is the primary means of changing aggressive behavior toward peers.[32]

One final, but important, caveat on using mediation and negotiation between bullies and targets. Some children who participate in bullying behaviors do so not as a primary instigator but as an "egger-on" or tangential support system for the bully himself. These children may be very responsive to both discipline and mediation, at least during elementary school years. They typically underestimate the destructiveness of their own behaviors, even when they themselves have been bullied (Elizabeth K. Englander. Coping with aggression and bullying as a teacher [personal communication, Massachusetts Aggression Reduction Center, Bridgewater State College, Bridgewater, MA, 2004]). If a school is able to identify a child as an "egger" rather than as a full-fledged bully, negotiations, mediations, or apologies may be effective during the elementary school years.

Responding to cyberbullying can be tricky as well. Unlike traditional bullying, cyberbullying frequently takes place off campus, most typically in the child's home. The fact that cyberbullying takes place predominantly off campus means that the behavior potentially falls into a different legal category. Whereas behavior that takes

Table 1	
Action steps to take in cyberbullying cases	
Have an educational discussion with the cyberbully and with cyber-bystanders.	It may be important to point out that this discussion is not discipline; it is educational, about the dangers of cyberbullying and the fact that everyone is now aware of the situation. If relevant, discuss future legal problems the child may incur if they continue with these behaviors. You can involve an School Resource Officer (SRO) or other police officer in the discussion, and the child's parents, if possible.
Immediately inform cyberbullies and cyber-bystanders about the consequences for bullying or cyberbullying in school.	If the cyberbully or cyber-bystanders engage in any bullying or cyberbullying in school, follow through on consequences immediately.
Be sure that a victim has a Safety and Comfort Plan.	This should include a Safe Person in school—someone who the child likes and can go to, and the child's teachers must be told that this child has the freedom to go see their Safe Person at any time. Initially, do not be concerned if a victim seems to exploit their Safe Person as a way to avoid schoolwork. Focus instead on the child's sense of safety and comfort. Eventually, when the situation seems to be resolved, you can address a child who exploits the situation (if necessary).
Inform all relevant adults	Inform teachers, coaches, counselors, and bus drivers about the situation between the 2 children. Ensure that they are aware of the potential for bullying and that they keep a very sharp eye open.
Have a plan for less structured areas, such as buses and lunchroom.	The victim should never be left to hope that they find a safe seat.
Follow-up with parents, especially parents of victims.	Do not wait for them to call you; call them to let them know that these actions are being taken.

place on the school campus is clearly under the jurisdiction of educators, behavior that takes place at home is usually viewed as being under the jurisdiction of parents.

However, even if a school decides that cyberbullying is not within the school's jurisdiction, there are still important steps (**Table 1**) that all schools can make to help cope with and resolve cyberbullying incidents.

How is the MARC Different from Other Centers and How Can Its Model be Replicated Elsewhere?

In the fall of 2004, I began a year as the first Presidential Fellow at Bridgewater State College in Bridgewater, Massachusetts. That year was utilized to set up the MARC and launch its model programs to the Massachusetts K to 12 educational community.

The approach of the Center is somewhat different from that of most other experts and centers in the field of bullying prevention. First, the center is an academic center, with a salaried faculty member as its director. It brings services to K to 12 education at either no cost or a very low cost to schools. This has removed the necessity of charging high fees from a field of expertise that previously was largely defined by the marketplace. In addition, MARC utilizes the resources of an academic institution in a very efficient manner. Services from the center are provided by faculty members, graduate students, and trained undergraduates. The undergraduates in the center are particularly valuable as high-status role-model peers in helping teenagers in local high schools form and promote their own bullying prevention work in their own schools.

When MARC goes into a school, we focus not only on services but on assistance with the implementation of services.[33] While assisting schools with implementation, we work intensively with administrators, classroom teachers, support staff, students, and parent and community groups. We have found that it is critical to address both bullying and cyberbullying; to only address traditional bullying is, in effect, to miss half the lesson. Several issues demand a particular focus when doing cyberbullying and bullying prevention work in K to 12 schools.

Be Up-to-Date Regarding Information Technology and Its Misuses

This is not a reference to traditional knowledge about computers; knowing how to use Excel or Google is not enough. What are the problems that are currently referenced on security blogs? What trends in cyber behavior are currently seen? What kinds of cyberbullying are kids engaging in? It is not enough to know that kids can send each other nasty e-mails.

Understand that Cyberbullying and Bullying are Different but Not Separate

For the cyber immersion generation, cyberbullying and bullying are integral and cannot be separated. If it happens in person, it will likely spill over into online life—and vice versa. Yet the causes of these 2 types of bullying are different. Despite that, the coexistence of these 2 worlds needs to be understood and expected.

Understand that the Role of Technology is Not Going Away

Using a "just turn it off" argument will only accomplish 1 result: Students will be certain that adults do not understand how they live and how they work. The cyber world is here to stay. Preparing children to live online may seem like a waste of time, unless you consider the alternative.

Education About Cyberbullying is an Important Part of Internet Safety

Many schools see Internet safety as a separate issue from cyberbullying, but children are much more likely to be cyberbullied than they are to be stalked or approached online by a threatening adult.[34]

We Must Begin Talking with Children About Cyberlife and How It Fits in with "Real" Life

The only safety mechanism that children will ultimately retain is the one between their ears. Yet most parents and most schools do not discuss Internet safety and cyberbullying with children. As cited, 1 study found that a mere 8% of schools in the United States have any education for children about Internet safety or bullying, even though experts agree that education in this area is the key to safety.[35]

Encouraging Reporting is Job One

Although many educators are very good at encouraging reporting, this is an issue where there is always room for improvement. It is through these connections between students and adults where targets will be best able to cope with bullying and where bullies themselves may learn about their own culpability in a safe environment.[a]

During its first several years, outcome data have identified several elements as the most important aspects of the MARC program.

Element 1: Acknowledge that educators are overwhelmed, cannot know everything, and offer them help with implementation and assistance

There is no real substitute for an in-depth knowledge of the realities of teaching today. Factors such as low pay, tenure, the pressures of standardized testing, and increased class size may seem unrelated to bullying, but in fact they are quite important. Increasing the pressure on teachers to be up to date in their fields decreases the time they have to gain expertise in new fields (such as cyberbullying). Acknowledging these realities renders classroom teachers and support staff more willing and ready to acquire new skills and be more receptive to the source of new information. In-service trainings, where expertise is brought to the school to train its faculty, must be responsive to the taxed and overwhelmed state of mind most educators bring to the training. Asking these professionals, for example, to explore their own personal feelings publicly may be well-intentioned, but often seem to be interpreted as a waste of time; no one is really receptive to enforced psychotherapy under the guise of education. In contrast, emphasizing very practical and concrete steps that teachers can take away and implement immediately can actively encourage their acceptance of effective interventions.

Cyberbullying education for faculty needs to focus on the 6 issues noted. The goal is not just to make sure that faculty have a sense of "what is happening out there," but also to raise their awareness about the difference between their use of the Internet and their students'. Such awareness is truly the first step to understanding and discussions with children.

Because bullying and cyberbullying are so enmeshed, we rarely address 1 issue without addressing the other. Concrete response skills are an important element in changing the culture of a school: What should a teacher do when encountering, for example, a student who seems to be the victim of bullying, but insists that it is just "fooling around"? These are the kinds of concrete issues, in addition to online problems, that need to be addressed for schoolteachers and staff in schools today. Space limitations here prevent a complete review of the issues and examples we use, but our website has more information (available at: www.MARCcenter.org).

Element 2: Use of the academic/teaching model rather than the marketplace model

An academic center reduces and scales costs, removes the profit motive by utilizing a salaried professor as a director, utilizes existing resources very effectively (such as students, computer and physical infrastructure, high-quality levels of knowledge and expertise), and establishes, for the schools seeking services, a dependable source of qualified professionals. Using academic experts is no panacea and their knowledge

---

[a]Encouraging reporting by children should be a high priority for every single principal in elementary, middle, junior, or high schools. In every single school shooting studied by the Secret Service (2002)[36], other children knew about the shooting before the actual event but did not report it to adults. It is no exaggeration to state that encouraging reporting—especially in middle, junior, and high schools—can literally save lives.

about children's aggression and bullying may not always be as high quality as desired, but academia generally represents a more dependable source of expertise than that offered by the public marketplace.

Element 3: Research-informed practice
What works with bullies? What types of adult responses actually reduce their abusive behaviors? What do we know about the difference between different types of bullies (eg, "bullies" versus "only-cyberbullies"). Research on traditional bullying abounds, although paucity characterizes the body of research on cyberbullying. Nevertheless, informed practices are best practices and it is important to keep in touch with the difference between anecdotal and experimental evidence—however compelling anecdotal evidence in the field may be.

Element 4: Distinction between bullying and conflict
The final research element is the recognition that bullying and conflict are not the same. Bullying, unlike conflict, is defined by a power differential: A bully is very powerful, whereas a victim has little or no social power in the situation.[37] This power differential means that, unlike equal power conflicts, the bully has little or no incentive to "settle" the conflict; rather, he or she may be invested in its continuation.[38] This is an important reason to avoid mediating bullying conflicts, because successful mediation requires both parties to have some motivation to end the conflict in question.[38]

Element 5: Produce innovative programming that addresses persistent obstacles
First, adults need to become much more aware of the difference between the generations—the cyber utilization versus the cyber immersion generations. Second, the most up-to-date issues emerging in cyberspace should be reviewed. Third, adults need guidance on beginning conversations with children about cyberbullying and cybersafety. The second issue renders long-term research difficult regarding outcomes, because no cyberbullying program can or should remain static for 3 or more years—the field itself evolves much more rapidly and our curricula is updated monthly to reflect that. (This is not an argument that outcomes research should not occur; it is merely an acknowledgement of the difficulty faced in this area.)

Element 6: Address school climate
This means that everyone—faculty, administration, students, and parents—must get involved. Students, especially adolescent students, need to be proactive partners, not passive recipients of adult-led programs. Adults need to be sensitized to the issue of cyberbullying, to the reality of the school day, to the limitations schools face, and to their own responsibilities at home and in the community. It is easy to list these issues and very difficult to achieve them. Despite the obvious implication of current statistics, we have encountered a staggering number of educators who deny the existence of any cyberbullying in "their" schools entirely. Parents, similarly, are often completely unaware of what their child is doing online (and sometimes in person) and, in any case, engaging their interest and attendance is a struggle. Innovative methods need to be found. We have experimented with morning presentations, evening presentations, parent/child discussion homework assignments, and local cable access TV and generally find that each method reaches a different subset of the community. This probably means that multiple efforts must be made at every school, but the future growth of the Internet may be 1 good avenue for communication.

REFERENCES

1. Nansel TR, Overpeck M, Pilla RS, et al. Bullying behaviors among U.S. youth: Prevalence and association with psychosocial adjustment. JAMA 2001;285:2094–100.
2. Olweus D. Bullying at school: what we know and what we can do. Cambridge (MA): Blackwell Publishers, Inc; 1993.
3. Cohn A, Canter A. Bullying: facts for schools and parents. National Association of School Psychologists; 2003. Available at: http://www.naspcenter.org/resources. Accessed June 29, 2007.
4. Englander E. Bullying and cyberbullying in Massachusetts today: recent research findings. Presented at the Annual Meeting of the Massachusetts Association of Colleges For Teacher Education. Sturbridge (MA), April 15, 2011:
5. Englander E. Cyberbullying: the new frontier. Proceedings of the Twenty-Third Annual Pediatric Rehabilitation Conference. Franciscan Hospital for Children and Boston University School of Medicine. Burlington (MA), March 23, 2007.
6. US Department of Education, National Center for Education Statistics. The continuation of Education, NCES 2002-025. Washington, DC: US Government Printing Office; 2002. Available at: http://nces.ed.gov. Accessed September 20, 2011.
7. National Education Association. National bullying awareness campaign; 2003. Available at: www.nea.org/schoolsafety/bullying.html. Accessed July 24, 2007.
8. National School Safety and Security Services. School deaths, school shootings, and high-profile incidents of school violence; 2005. Available at: http://www.schoolsecurity.org/trends/school_violence.html. Accessed July 24, 2007.
9. National Youth Violence Prevention Resource Center. Facts for teens; 2002. Available at: http://www.safeyouth.org. Accessed July 30, 2006.
10. Englander E. Exposure to violence can have significant impact on children." [Op-Ed]. Brockton Sunday Enterprise. September 30, 2001.
11. Olweus D. Bully/victim problems among school children: Some basic facts and effects of a school based intervention Program. In: Pepler D, Rubin K, editors. The development and treatment of childhood aggression. Hillsdale (NJ): Erlbaum; 1991. p. 411–38.
12. Davis S. Schools where everyone belongs: Practical strategies for reducing bullying. Wayne (ME): Research Press; 2004.
13. LaHoud S. Bridgewater State professor takes aim at bullying. Attleboro Sun Chronicle. March 18, 2007.
14. Brown J, Cassidy. Cyber-bullying: developing policy to direct responses that are equitable and effective in addressing this special form of bullying. Canadian Journal of Educational Administration and Policy 2006;57:8–11.
15. Pew Internet & American Life Project. "Cyberbullying and online teens; 2007. Available at: http://www.pewinternet.org/PPF/r/216/report_display.asp. Accessed July 31, 2007.
16. Englander E. Spare the bully and spoil the school. Presented at the National Trends in Violence Prevention Conference. Topsfield (MA). March 22, 2006.
17. Englander E, Lawson C. Bullies, eggers, and bystanders: new approaches to preventing peer abuse among children. In: Terr LC, Webb NB, editors. Play therapy with children in crisis. 3rd edition. New York: Guilford Press; 2007. pp. 37–56.
18. Aftab P. WiredSafety. Irvington-on-Hudson, NY: Wired Kids, Inc.; 2005. Available at: http://wiredsafety.org. Accessed July 3, 2007.
19. Staub E. Aggression and self-esteem. APA Monitor Online; 1999, January 1. Available at: http://www.apa.org/monitor/jan99/point.html. Accessed July 18, 2007.

20. Kruger J, Epley N, Parker J, et al. Egocentrism over e-mail: can we communicate as well as we think? J Personality Soc Psychol 2005;89:925–36.
21. Stevahn, L. Integrating conflict resolution and peer mediation training into the curriculum. Theory Into Practice 2004;43(1):50–8.
22. Burrell N, Zirbel C, Allen M. Evaluating peer mediation outcomes in educational settings. Conflict Resolution Quarterly 2003;21(1):7–26.
23. Rubin R. Building a comprehensive discipline system and strengthening school climate. Reclaiming Children and Youth 2004;13(3):162–9.
24. Casella R. The benefits of peer mediation in the context of urban conflict and program status. Urban Education 2000;35(3)324–55.
25. Theberge SK, Karan O. Six factors inhibiting the use of peer mediation in a junior high school. Professional School Counseling 2004;7(4):283–6.
26. Delisio ER. Making peer mediation a part of campus life. 2004. Available at: http://www.education-world.com/a_admin/admin/admin348.shtml. Accessed August 27, 2011.
27. Adams RJ. Awesome talking library: bullying basics;2004. available at: http://www.awesomelibrary.org/bullying.html. Accessed August 27, 2011.
28. Englander EK. Understanding violence. 2nd edition. Mahwah (NJ): Lawrence Erlbaum and Associates, Publishers; 2003.
29. Dodge KA, Lansford JE, Salzer Burks V, et al. Peer rejection and social information-processing factors in the development of aggressive behavior problems in children. Child Development 2003;74(2):374–93.
30. Johnson D, Lewis G. Do you like what you see? Self-perceptions of adolescent bullies. British Educational Research Journal 1999;25(5):19–26.
31. Bluestein J. Creating emotionally safe schools. Deerfield Beach (FL): Health Communications, Inc; 2001.
32. Olweus D. Bullying at school: what we know and what we can do. Cambridge (MA): Blackwell; 1993.
33. Berends M, Bodilly S, Kirby SN. Facing the challenges of whole-school reform: new American schools after a decade. Santa Monica, CA: The Rand Corporation; 2002.
34. Bangeman E. Study: fears over kid's online safety overblown; 2007. Available at: http://arstechnica.com/news.ars. Accessed August 9, 2007.
35. Devaney L. Education the key to better security; 2007. Available at: http://www.eschoolnews.com/news/showStory.cfm?ArticleID=7253. Accessed July 31, 2007.
36. The final report and findings of the safe school initiative: implications for the prevention of school attacks in the United States. Available at: http://www.secretservice.gov/ntac/ssi_final_report.pdf. Washington, DC: US Secret Service and US Department of Education; 2002.
37. Vaillancourt T. Toward a bully-free community: the case of Hamilton, Ontario, Canada. Teaching and Learning 2004;1(3):14–6.
38. Englander E. When should you hesitate to mediate? Models of Respecting Everyone 2005;1(1):2–5.

When a Student Dies: Organizing the School's Response

Mike S. Jellinek, MD*, Uchenwa D. Okoli, MD

KEYWORDS

• Crisis counseling • Death • Grief • School

Principals, teachers, and guidance counselors feel ill-prepared to address a student's death. Often the death is not anticipated, comes as a shock, and has many reverberations in the school itself and in the broader community. Students die from multiple causes including accidents, suicide, homicide, or chronic illness; leading causes of death may vary depending on age group. The principal and others in the school may be called upon to serve as leaders in this sudden crisis and have broad responsibilities to their school community that may seem overwhelming in the face of their own grief and reactions to the loss. These guidelines present a meaningful response to an event that can profoundly affect the school and community.

INITIAL RESPONSE: THE CRISIS TEAM

A crisis team is a good starting point for planning communication.[1] The goal of the crisis team is restore equilibrium in school community, and help to instill a sense of safety, connectedness, and hope.[2] The core team usually consists of the principal (the team leader), assistant principal, school psychologist/social worker, guidance counselor, and 1 or 2 senior teachers. (In cases of complex emotional circumstances, a consulting child psychiatrist may be helpful; in a gang-related homicide, the local police commander may be key, and in a broader disaster, an experienced member of the Red Cross is often a valued addition). Include school nurses early in the planning process[3] or add them to the team as there may be medical information to assess as well as the infirmary becoming a focal point for vulnerable students. This team crafts the initial announcement; decides how to disseminate information, and alerts essential staff regarding schedule changes, meetings, setting up a crisis center, and so on. Initial planning may be as simple a communication strategy, or it may be more complex if there is a threat of ongoing danger, multiple deaths, or public health concerns. If the deceased student's siblings attend other schools in the community, the crisis team should advise their principals. The crisis team is instrumental in delegating responsibilities individual members, helping to maintain structure and order, while minimizing any confusion of roles. The team may assign roles to

Department of Psychiatry, Massachusetts General Hospital, Harvard Medical School, Newton, MA, USA
* Corresponding author.
E-mail address: mjellinek@partners.org

Child Adolesc Psychiatric Clin N Am 21 (2012) 57–67
doi:10.1016/j.chc.2011.08.008
1056-4993/12/$ – see front matter © 2012 Elsevier Inc. All rights reserved.

Box 1
Crisis team major responsibilities

- Confirm identity of student, verify details of the death, contact family of the deceased, and discuss information family will disclose to school community.
- Coordinate internal and external resources: Activate phone tree to alert crisis members, and designate roles to facilitate quick decision making and needed liaisons (eg, media, police, parent-teacher organization).
- Inform school board and administration of student death. Construct a concise written statement to share with students, teachers, and parents.
- Contact feeder or receiver schools so that they can provide support for students affected in their schools.
- Media liaison to make press release or schedule a press conference.
- Arrange first faculty meeting before or after school.
- Collect deceased students' belongings from his/her locker.
- Assess needs for homeroom meetings and prepare discussion points for teachers to review with students. Teachers make adjustments to schedule (eg, postpone testing and shorten assignments) to accommodate needs of students.
- Assess impact on all school events such as varsity sports and other extracurricular activities.
- Identify high-risk staff and students in need of counseling, initiate groups for the victim's friends; conduct posttraumatic loss debriefings to deal with posttraumatic effects of the loss. Consider designating a care center away from office for students who need additional time to cope with situation.
- Provide that support personnel be available for emergency counseling with students or faculty after hours.
- Provide any needed security for school building or students.
- Follow-up specifically with the faculty or school staff directly involved in the crisis and conduct regular debriefing sessions with them.
- Distribute list of community resources to professionals and parents, such as mental health providers, parent support groups.
- Express appreciation to all persons who helped handle the crisis.
- During the acute stabilization phase, continue to
- Keep administration and counseling staff informed of any problems. Provide staff with daily briefings, consider before and after school faculty meetings, issue daily written updates for staff and parents.
- Debrief counseling staff at beginning and end of the day.
- Focus on the needs of survivors and continue to identify high-risk students and staff who would benefit from counseling services.
- Call parents of students counseled to provide continued support for the students who are unusually distressed.
- Assess acuity of crisis in school community, and ongoing need for crisis team. Consider plans for demobilization when appropriate.
- During extended stabilization phase, consider
- Using standing groups to plan for faculty meetings, any expected impact to academic program, and if there needs to be a longer term process to reassess school values.
- Reviewing guidelines for short term memorials and if any longer plan memorial group will be formed. Remain alert for any grief reactions that may result owing to anniversaries of student's death.

Adapted from Thompson R. Being prepared for suicide or sudden death in schools: strategies to restore equilibrium. J Mental Health 1995;17:264.

---

individual team members, for example, media liaison, and community liaison, security liaison in effort to facilitate timely decision making.[4] An overview of the crisis team's role is provided in **Box 1.**

The initial demand is often for information. Given the use of cell phones and texting, there are often facts and rumors spreading far and wide within minutes of the death.

The crises team should gather initial information about the death and in a thoughtful and circumspect manner release a statement on what is known. If there is any early contact or access to the family (usually through a trusted teacher or parent), reviewing any information that is about to be released should be part of the plan. The focus of the communication with students and staff should be strictly factual, not speculative. Acknowledging exactly what is unknown is better than trying to fill in the gaps. To forestall possible negative behaviors, the message should be empathic to student's likely feelings. For example, the crisis team may acknowledge that some students may feel very depressed or even feel that life is not worth living after the loss of a friend as part of offering meeting places and counseling services. Another example would be to acknowledge that after the death of a student passenger in a car accident, some may wish to retaliate against the driver of the car or the driver who precipitated the accident. The communication should suggest ways that staff members and students can address their concerns, include a promise for ongoing communication, offer a place to meet and discuss the issues as well as encourage questions and feedback. It often lowers anxiety to let the community know when the next communication will be issued (often a schedule of 3 specific times a day makes sense) rather than everyone waiting indefinitely. The initial announcement should be a written statement that is provided to teachers, parents, students, and media outlets allowing for unified, consistent transmission of information and to minimize any confusion.

If off hours, it is preferable to notify staff members individually, perhaps through the faculty phone chain, to allow them initial privacy to contend with the death. The crisis team can then meet with faculty members or with the entire faculty, who typically need to address their own reactions before meeting with classes of students. The principal or school counselor should lead any meeting and avoid making announcements in too large an assembly or over a public address system. Scheduling a faculty meeting before and after school for the first several days can help to monitor the school community by listening to the faculty's feedback, answer the many questions, and provide support to the faculty directly. Although individuals may have strong personal reactions, the faculty group will have added balancing and supportive comments. Early on the crisis team also plays a key role with identifying individual students in need of support,[4] generally, students who were friends of the deceased, who had any involvement in the circumstances of the death, who may identify closely, or are currently suffering from depression.

INFLUENCE OF SOCIAL NETWORKING

Social networking plays an increasingly large role in how quickly information is transmitted about recent events in real time. School-age children often have access to cell phones, Twitter, and Facebook, increasing the ability to communicate in seconds. Social media plays a large role in keeping students connected and abreast of tragic situations such as a student death. Students may turn to the internet as an outlet for their grief.[5] In a survey of 203 students involved in 2007 mass homicide shootings of Virginia Tech and Northern Illinois University, 89% joined at least one Facebook group concerning the shooting, 64% had left message concerning the shooting on someone's wall, 78% used an on-line chat program to discuss the shooting (such as AOL Instant Messenger), and 74% had used text messaging.[5] Students may opt to memorialize the deceased by creating on-line groups or updating their status to reflect the student's death. Many students interpret these social media connections as supportive and positive.[5] However, risks are also involved with quick transmission of information, especially when inaccurate, unconfirmed details about student death, quickly become "viral." Thus, it is important that the crisis team is quickly involved with of spread of accurate information with students and staff to limit rumors and transmission of false information. The crisis team may ask 1 of its members to track some of the social media sites to assess the quality of the information and any worrisome comments or trends. If not possible to assess directly, guidance counselors may be able to get information from students using the sites.

HOW THE SCHOOL AND STUDENTS REACT

The needs of students and staff members depends on their relationship to the deceased, their coping mechanisms, and the circumstances surrounding the death.[6]

Student Reactions

A large percentage of students will be affected by the loss of a peer. Initially, the deceased student's closest friends need support from a school counselor. The school might offer students repeated opportunities to talk together, offer group lunches or meetings after school. If several students were directly exposed to the accident or suicide, they may benefit from group opportunities to discuss their reactions. For example, after a bus accident, the surviving students met as a group with a skilled child psychiatrist before facing their peers and the press. Students with a history of trauma and loss (eg, the death of a parent) or with a history of depression or other mood disorders require frequent monitoring. In 1 circumstance on which we were consulted, a classmate was particularly distraught after a 13-year-old girl died of cancer. A guidance counselor learned that this classmate's mother had died of breast cancer 3 years earlier. The guidance counselor sought the student out and contacted the family to alert them to the likely rekindling of grief and to the warning signs of depression.

Students and faculty respond on their own time lines, and therefore the individual pace of denial, anger, and despondency or acceptance varies widely.[7] As a result, school administrators must rely on students and staff as daily barometers to help them monitor how rapidly the school should resume a regular routine and how much time students and staff need collectively to grieve the loss. Of course, individual students may need an extended period; generally, restoring routines and structure of school helps the grieving process. A return to classes, homework, and routine activities is usually indicated within a few days.[8]

Survivors each experience the loss in a different way, with unanticipated emotions often overwhelming their rational understanding of death. Typically:

- Preschool students are involved with magical thinking, and have little understanding about the permanence of death. They may seem to be "casual" or excited about rituals surrounding death.
- Elementary students worry most about the effect of the death on their immediate lives; they tend to benefit from the reassurance that they are safe and their family will not substantially change.
- Middle grades students are usually concerned about how they might have foreseen or even prevented this death, so they may benefit from a discussion of the facts surrounding the death and a clarification of their lack of responsibility (usually) in the death.
- High school students often worry about the finality of this person's death, and probably benefit most from a discussion of the meaning of the student's life and what will persist after the funeral.

Students very close to the deceased or feeling profound guilt that they should have recognized suicidal intent or stopped a friend from driving after drinking are at special risk. Survivors have varied reactions and behaviors in response to student's death. It is important to monitor closely for any maladaptive coping behaviors including worsening mood symptoms, substance abuse, social isolation, and oppositional behavior.[4] The crisis team should arrange for the availability of mental health resources to provide for students and families.

Staff Reactions

Staff reactions influence how teachers present information to students. An administrator or counselor should maintain ongoing communication with teachers and staff members who worked directly with the deceased student. This can help to clarify which staff members are having the most difficulty and suggest additional interventions. In 1 instance, a teacher was particularly overwhelmed when a student died in an alcohol-related traffic accident. When the principal reached out to speak with him, the teacher described the family history of alcoholism that contributed to his brother's death in a car accident many years before the current incident. The principal was then able to understand the teacher's reaction and encourage outside counseling so the teacher could separate, and address, both events. In another circumstance, a teacher had arranged most appropriately for a school group to visit another school. The bus crashed and several students were killed. The teacher's guilt, despite not being the driver, being hurt himself, and simply doing his job, was profound.

Parents' Reactions

Parents often worry about their child's psychological and emotional reaction to a death in the school community. If a student died owing to homicide, they may worry of their child's safety in that particular school. Having a member of the police force on the crisis team in this circumstance is critical. Parents may feel helpless and attempt to find ways to help staff and students at school with coping. They may call the school inquiring about any updates, or volunteer to help on the crisis team. It is important that the school maintain ongoing, predictable communications with parents, updating them with any relevant information. Parent meetings and using the communication pathways of the parent-teacher organization is often helpful. Schools may also create a parent hot line number where any updates may be obtained. Of course, parents should be key monitors of their own child's reaction and be urged to contact guidance personnel if they have any concerns. The head of the parent-teacher organization is an appropriate liaison to the crisis team (although probably should not be a member; the team should be composed of school staff and any needed consultant). Over time, the parent-teacher organization can help to arrange parent meetings and outside speakers to help process the loss.

WHY AND WHO'S TO BLAME?

The death of a child or adolescent unleashes strong emotions. People often try to soothe themselves by searching for answer or relief from the feelings of loss and risk. Many find temporary relief by focusing intense feelings of anxiety, blame, anger, and guilt in the form of attack on some individual thought to be responsible. The tone and content of communication from the crisis team can anticipate some of these reactions and redirect students, families, and school staff back to grieving and reasonable discussion of life's risks. Often, the crisis team is a microcosm of the range of feelings in the school and in the community. The team's discussions and coming to a reasonable consensus often helps to find the right wording, timing, and emphasis that shape the teams recommendations and actions.

Accidents

Accidents are the leading cause of death in young people of children and young adults, resulting in 43% of deaths in this age group.[9] Accidents are particularly difficult because of their suddenness, but also because o the perception that someone might have been able to prevent them. Blame may settle on a teacher who did not notify the principal's office about a student who skipped a class and later died in a car accident. People may blame other students who survived the accident but encouraged the driver to skip, drink, or look away from the road. In accidents in which some students survive and others do not, educators should anticipate and attempt to prevent students from taking action against surviving students out of misguided loyalty.[10] This is particularly important given the increased risk of violence in students who have been bullied in school.[11] In such cases, schools need to indicate to students how they may express their loyalty in more meaningful ways.

Clinical example

In the bus crashed mentioned, several families were involved in arranging funerals. Each was of a different religion and had differing wishes. The crisis team had liaisons to each family, communicated their wishes in 1 of the 3-a-day communications bulletins, and organized the customized school response to each funeral.

To cope with the many students, teachers, family members, friends, and members of the community who wanted and needed to come together, a large ceremony was arranged under a tent in the school playground, which was attended by over 1500persons. Each family arranged for their own memorial and the school had a stone etched with an image and each child's name that was inserted as part of the school building.

Suicide

Suicides are the third leading cause of death in young people of children and young adults.[9] The suicide of a child or adolescent occurs more frequently during the spring semester.[12] Because details of the suicide frequently become a focus of attention, it is important to provide brief, accurate information that has been cleared with the family (eg, "Tracy died from a gunshot wound"). Posing such questions as, "What do you think Tracy would want us to be talking about?" or "How will it be helpful for us to talk about these details?" can redirect students' efforts to obtain more details or personal information. Those close to the student often believe that they missed or failed to respond to signs from the student. In addition, faculty and students often believe they may have said or done something that contributed to the suicidal act (eg, assigning too much homework).

Bullying has gained increased attention in recent years, as social media has covered high-profile cases of students involved with school bullying and death. Youth who are bullied, or who bully others, are at an elevated risk for suicidal thoughts, attempts, and completion.[13] Often, students who complete suicide have other, often private, emotional and psychological issues. Social networking has gained increased attention with its role in cyber-bulling, which is also related to increased suicidal ideation.[14] Clearly, a suicide complicated by cyber-bullying is a crisis involving many students and the culture of the school that did not protect its students. The cultural issues frequently included distrust with faculty groups or with the school administration and difficulties among the faculty in accepting responsibility and sharing similar values. The cultural and community ramifications require a program, sometimes a year long, to foster healing.

The anger after a suicide is frequently displaced from the victim toward other students or staff,[15] increasing the likelihood of assaults or additional incidents of students harming themselves. Contacting students close to the victim and examining their reactions privately may reveal the role they perceive themselves to have played in the suicide or any thoughts they may harbor about engaging in self-destructive behavior out of loyalty to the victim. A suicide also increases the risk of self-destructive behavior in those suffering from depression or who have attempted suicide in the past.[16] The closeness of the suicide makes the act a more realistic option in the minds of some adolescents. Some students, especially those feeling unpopular or isolated, may be drawn to suicide because of the community reaction, which can seem to glorify the deceased student. Guidance counselors often feel under pressure to prevent to contagion of suicide and monitor all the vulnerable students. In a high school of 1000 adolescents, statistically 100 or more are particularly vulnerable. It is helpful to tell the guidance counselor staff the truth: Predicting suicide is practically impossible; the most school counselors can do is monitor the students at risk, provide support and a sense of connection, and refer those most in need to local services. The guidance counselor group needs support because they are expected (and burdened) to try and prevent another attempted of completed suicide.

Clinical example
A senior who had dedicated much of his life to getting into a very competitive college was terribly disappointed that he had been rejected. Although many knew that getting into this college was very important to him, no one saw him as depressed or at risk for harming himself, especially given his other options. The day after the rejection, this senior went home and committed suicide by handgun. The school community was thunderstruck and long-simmering tensions in the school and in the community came to the fore. How important is getting into a name college? Was there too much competition? Why did not anyone know this young man was at risk? Were we assigning too much homework? Grading too hard or not hard enough? The splits within the faculty made the school setting feel unstable and not a cultural structure that could contain the many emotions of the adolescents wrestling with this suicide and the associated anxiety/loss.

Two large, all-faculty meetings were called on successive days and then a follow-up meeting a week later. These meetings were used by the crisis team to communicate with teachers, scan for students and teachers at risk, discuss a brief homeroom curriculum to support students, arrange for faculty–student lunches, and to have extended discussions about the schools values, standards, parental pressures, faculty tensions, and to discuss the complexities/limitations of suicide prediction. Over the 3 meetings, many faculty and administrative tensions were unearthed and the principal set forth a work plan for a newly named committee of faculty leaders. The faculty came together in affirming the value of their academic approach (pending committee review) and accepted that predicting suicide was both beyond their responsibility and, in fact, not possible in a group of high-functioning, not depressed teenagers. As the faculty came together, within hours the tension level in school eased with more open grieving, discussion, and planning.

Homicide

Homicide is the second leading cause death among children and adolescents between 10 and 24 years old.[9] It is leading cause of death for African Americans between ages 15 and 24 years.[9] School-associated homicides are very rare, and make up less than 1% of homicides that occur among school-aged youths.[17] In a review of 116 school-associated homicides from July 1999 to June 2006, 65% resulted from gunshot wounds, 27% stabbing or cutting, and 12% beatings.[17] Despite reports in the media, the incidence of individual events with mass student homicides, for example, Columbine High School in 1999, are rare. Homicides in a school setting are a fearful experience. Students may also display symptoms of trauma after a school shooting.[18] Teachers and students must learn to cope with the violence-related crisis. Students may feel unsafe and helpless on school grounds, uncertain if additional violence will result in retaliation to homicide. If a student witnessed a shooting, they may be afraid to report the assailant to the authorities. Police officers may increase their presence in the school setting. Parents may express concern about their child's safety on school grounds. It is important for the crisis team to be actively involved in communication with students and parents in an effort to provide reassurance and comfort. After the crisis phase, these events require a community-wide program, lasting months to years, to reestablish a communities' sense of emotional integrity.

Chronic Illness

Cancer is the fourth leading cause of death in children and young adults ages 1 to 24 years old; however, it is the second leading cause in children ages 5 to 14 years old.[9] Chronic illness resulting a student's death is sometimes less traumatic to a school, particularly if surviving students were prepared and had opportunities to say good-bye. Still, some staff members and students may not have believed that the students would really die; they may feel cheated by God because their prayers went unanswered. Students of all ages sometimes fear they might "catch" whatever caused the chronic illness and then feel guilty for having avoided the student. Discussions should acknowledge student guilt and fears, as well as address how people can contend with severe or chronic illnesses.[7]

Student deaths from chronic illness are often more difficult for adults, who experience a different version of survivor guilt as they question the meaning of death for someone who will never experience the joys of childhood or adulthood. Such adults may need help recollecting the joys the dying student already has experienced; focusing on the joys the student can still experience while he or she is sufficiently healthy (eg, Make-A-Wish programs), and recognizing that these students may not have "missed" certain joys that they never thought about.

THE TIMETABLE OF GRIEF

Grieving is a process, not an event.[19] Unfortunately, administrators may sometimes prematurely attempt to reestablish the normal routine. This often comes off as lacking compassion, so it is helpful for administrators to talk with those who knew the student best to assess the mood of the school. Teachers may need to reassess expectations for completion of homework assignments and school absences. Staffing a designated room with clinical personnel can be helpful for at least 5 days after the death; schools sometimes decide to stay open on the first weekend after the death to provide a supervised place for those who wish to gather.

Schools should also provide a book in a designated office where students can come in and write to the deceased's family. This is preferable to placing pictures or newspaper articles about the death in prominent places where students must confront their feelings every time they walk by. Such a book should usually be available to students for about 4 weeks. Appropriate staff members can monitor writings to ensure they will be helpful to the family and to spot students who may be experiencing more-than-usual difficulty with the death. Similarly, encouraging a student to commemorate loss through some form of participation, such as drawing pictures or planting a tree, promotes inclusion in the process and provides a meaning ritual.[20]

Because it is normal to respond to an overwhelming event, posttraumatic debriefing should be available between 24 and 72 hours after the event. One should never force a discussion, but rather provide open conversation and exploration of the powerful feelings that shared traumatic events create.

The crisis team should gather information from the faculty meetings, counseling staff, nurse, message book, parents association, and their own conversations. The team can then plan letter and e-mail communications to students, faculty, and parents regarding such matters as the school's schedule, funeral arrangements (cultural/religious issues, who should attend, logistics of a large funeral), memorials, and meetings.[21]

Someone on the crisis team also needs to take responsibility for managing the large number of well-intentioned parents, volunteers, and mental health experts who may come to the school to offer help. The designated person should organize the efforts so they are compatible with the crisis team's plans and check credentials of any grief counselors, thus maintaining quality control. Students need protection—at least at the school—from intrusions by the media and inquisitive others. It is generally best to use school staff and provide referral information to parents for counseling outside of school.

INITIAL AND LONG-TERM MEMORIALS

A memorial, the formal acknowledgement and lasting recognition of someone's death, is a vital aspect of how we grieve. Planning a memorial can productively channel energy, be profoundly educational, and communicate key values. The school should be aware that students may experience grief reactions on crisis anniversaries (eg, after a month or a year after the death), and have adequate preparations in place to support students and staff.

The crisis team should define the location and likely duration of the initial memorial. For example, having flowers and notes at the school entrance, alerting students that the press will have access to the memorial outside the school (not inside), and deciding how long the memorial will stay in place (usually several days) help to organize students and staff. It is common for students within minutes to memorialize the deceased student's locker and desk using notes, drawings, flowers, and pictures. The principal should designate a site inside the building, such as a large bulletin board, for notes and pictures. The deceased student's locker and desk are often painful, personal sites, which after the first few days should be shifted so the halls and classroom can begin to return to functional status.

Clinical Example

After the unexpected death of a student with a chronic illness, the outpouring of emotion was overwhelming. Hundreds of flowers and notes virtually obstructed the hallway near her locker and her desk was surrounded by flowers in her classroom. There was a sense that nothing could be touched because it would be disrespectful and evoke much anger in the student body. The crisis team felt paralyzed; they want to resume classes. After extensive discussion within the team and with friends of the deceased, a compromise was communicated in the noon bulletin. The flowers would be removed over the weekend because they posed a health hazard. The notes would be removed and placed in a scrapbook available for viewing and additions in the main office. Given the 1 month of school left before summer vacation, the decorations on the locker door would be preserved and the desk and locker would not be reassigned until the next school year. Students had felt that they had not been able to control the uncontrollable loss of a beloved friend, dealt with that feeling by trying to control the memorial tinged with much anger. Once the crisis committee shared control with the students, they could give up some of the anger and experience sadness. Hundreds of students, taken by bus from the school to the chapel, attended the funeral.

The nature and placement of long-term memorials should be a thoughtful process. Placing permanent memorials in areas where they serve as constant reminders of the death can be problematic. Should students be reminded of a death every time they enter the school or eat lunch? Is there a place in the school where there are other memorials? It is often helpful for the principal or school counselor to meet with the deceased student's friends to talk about the scale and duration of memorials, especially if they are in public corridors or classrooms. Contact with the family to clarify and respect their wishes facilitates community cohesion.

Grieving students or faculty should take their time before deciding longer term memorials, such as scholarships. They need to address such questions as, How will we keep this student's name alive in the school? How will we honor this person's memory? What life lesson does this student's life—and death—provide? How can this death lead to expansion of helpful choices and guidance for future students? The most effective memorials connect generations of people by illuminating cherished principles or aspects of the deceased person's life that remain meaningful for us all.

DEMOBILIZING THE CRISIS TEAM

The school community may take weeks to months before a return to normalcy; however, the crisis team often begin to demobilize after community response procedures been concluded.[4] Crisis team members should have debriefing sessions to discuss reactions to student's death as responding may have caused compassion fatigue or resurfaced past losses.[4] Debriefing sessions are also helpful to evaluate the crisis team's overall performance and discuss what went well and what did not.

WHAT WE CAN LEARN

Each tragic death offers a window into the school's culture. Any problem in that school community—a poor relationship between faculty and administration or too much emphasis on a single aspect of the school's goals (eg, on academics or sports)—will come to the fore and complicate the school's coping with the death.

Each death also kindles a reexamination of the vital teachings and values of the school. This process should be embraced over the ensuing months with appropriate input from parents, students, faculty and administration. An anniversary ceremony is the final step in the recovery plan and reflects the school's reexamined and possibly evolved values in terms of remembering, repairing, preventing, and learning.

REFERENCES

1. Kline M, Schonfeld DJ, Lichtenstein R. Benefits and challenges of school-based crisis response teams. J School Health 1995;65:245–9.

2. Szumilas M, Wei Y, Kutcher K. Psychological debriefing in Schools. CMAJ 2010;182: 883–4.

3. Lohan JA. School nurses' support for bereaved students: a pilot study. J School Nurs 2006;22:48–52.

4. Streufert B. Death on campuses: common postvention strategies in higher education. Death Studies 2004;28:151–172.

5. Vicary A, Fraley R. Student reactions to the shootings at Virginia Tech and Northern Illinois University: does sharing grief and support over the internet affect recovery? Pers Soc Psychol Bull 2010;36:1555–1563.

6. Thompson R. Post-traumatic loss debriefing: providing immediate support for survivors of suicide or sudden loss. Ann Arbor, MI: ERIC Clearinghouse on Counseling and Personnel Services; 1990. (ERIC No. ED31570S). Available at: www.ericdigests.org/pre-9214/post.htm. Accessed August 23, 2011.

7. Ramer-Chrastek J. Hospice care for a terminally-ill child in the school setting. J School Nurs 2000;16:52–6.

8. Noppe LC, Noppe LD, Bartell D. Terrorism and resilience: adolescents' and teachers' responses to September 11, 2001. Death Studies 2006;30:41–60.

9. National Vital Statistics Report, 2005. Available at: http://www.cdc.gov/nchs/data/nvsr/nvsr54/nvsr54_02.pdf. Accessed August 23, 2011.

10. Twemlow SW, Fonagy P, Sacco FC, et al. Premeditated mass shootings in schools: threat assessment. J Am Acad Child Adolesc Psychiatry 2002;41:475–477.

11. Anderson M, Kaufman J, Simon TR, et al. School-associated violent deaths in the United States, 1994–1999. JAMA 2001;286:2695–702.

12. Temporal variations in school-associated student homicide and suicide events: United States, 1992–1999. Morbid Mortal Wkly Rep 2001;50:657–60. Available at: www.cdc.gov/mrmwr/preview/mmwrhtml/mm5031a1.htm. Accessed August 23, 2011.

13. Van der Wak MF, de Wit Cam, Hirasing RA. Psychological health among young victims and offenders of direct and indirect bullying. Pediatrics 2003;111:1312–7.

14. Hinduja S, Patchin JW. Bullying, cyberbullying, and suicide. Arch Suicide Res 2010; 14:206–21.

15. Newman EC. Group crisis intervention in a school setting following an attempted suicide. Int J Emerg Ment Health 2000;2:97–100.

16. Weinberger LE, Sreenivasan S, Sathyavagiswaran L, et al. Child and adolescent suicide in a large, urban area: psychological, demographic, and situational factors. J Forensic Sci 2001;46:902–7.

17. Centers for Disease Control and Prevention. Morbid Mortal Weekly Report 2007;57: 33–36. School-associated student homicides: United States, 1992–2006. Available at: http://www.cdc.gov/mmwr/preview/mmwrhtml/mm5702a1.htm. Accessed August 23, 2011.

18. Palinkas LA, Prussiing B, Reznik VM, et al. The San Diego East Country school shootings: a qualitative study of community level post-traumatic stress. Prehosp Disaster Med 2004;19:113–21.

19. Brock SE. Suicide postvention. Sacramento: California State University; 2001. Available at: www.csus.edu/indiv/b/brocks/Workshops/NASP/Suicide%20Postvention%20Paper.pdf. Accessed August 23, 2011.

20. Gibbons MB. A child dies, a child survives: the impact of sibling loss. J Pediatr Health Care 1992;6:65–72.

21. Berkowitz L, McCauley J, Schuurman DL, et al. Organizational postvention after Suicide death. In: Jordan JR, McIntosh JL, editors. Grief after suicide: understanding the consequences and caring for the survivors. New York: Routledge; 2010.

Building Better Brains: Evidence-Based Interventions to Enhance Contemporary Schooling

Jeffrey Q. Bostic, MD, EdD[a,b,*], Lauren J. Hart, BS[a,c]

KEYWORDS

• School • Mental health • Academic success

The vast majority of young people attend school. School provides a rich environment for cultivating academic skills such as reading, writing, and mathematics, but also for developing interpersonal skills, metacognitive skills such as executive functioning skills, and emotional regulation skills. The 15,000 hours most students spend in school are often guided by familiar but not evidence-based practices driven primarily to prepare students for antiquated needs rather than by contemporary findings about how the brain best learns and grows. Specifically, most schools still rely on a school day driven by previous social designs to prepare students for working on farms or in factories. The school day begins at sunup for most high school students despite clear evidence that adolescents require more sleep and stay up later because of biological changes surrounding puberty. Often, learning is still by rote methods, with a teacher-supervisor presenting information, then directing students to demonstrate understanding in the classroom and having them practice and extrapolate this learning independently at home. Although this approach may have some value and may be economical in terms of staff time, it is not predicated on emerging principles about how students best learn. In this article, biological conditions favorable to brain development, psychological skills associated with effective school functioning, and school practices associated with academic and interpersonal success are described so that schooling may increasingly be shaped more by brain development than social custom. Emerging findings about child development position child psychiatrists to influence school practices to better prepare children to enjoy their lives in the 21st century.

[a] Department of Psychiatry, Harvard Medical School, 6900 Yawkey Building, 55 Fruit Street, Boston, MA 02114, USA
[b] School Psychiatry, Massachusetts General Hospital, Boston, MA, USA
[c] Department of Public Health, Northeastern University, USA
* Corresponding author. Department of Child Psychiatry, 6900 Yawkey Building, 55 Fruit Street, Boston, MA 02114, USA
E-mail address: jbostic@partners.org

Child Adolesc Psychiatric Clin N Am 21 (2012) 69–80
doi:10.1016/j.chc.2011.09.006
1056-4993/12/$ – see front matter © 2012 Elsevier Inc. All rights reserved.
childpsych.theclinics.com

MODERN BIOLOGY AND SCHOOL PRACTICES

Advances in understanding of brain development and human growth have significant implications for school practices. Some of these findings provide support for previous educational practices, whereas others favor substantial departures from conventional school practices.

Nutrition, Obesity, and Exercise

The epidemic of obesity among young people requires different priorities within the school day. The availability of inexpensive but unhealthy foods and the increased frequency of eating throughout the school day of high-fat, low nutritive–value snacks contributes to unhealthy patterns of eating; because practice makes permanent, altering these unhealthy patterns becomes increasingly difficult the longer schools allow them.

Students consume a significant amount of their daily caloric intake at school. The National School Lunch Program served over 5 billion lunches, and the National School Breakfast Program served almost 2 billion breakfasts in 2010[1] not including snacks available to students through cafeterias and vending machines during and after school. Schools that participate in the National School Lunch or Breakfast Programs are required to follow nutritional guidelines.[1] Unhealthy foods are usually found in vending machines, and "the strongest risk factor for buying snacks or beverages from vending machines instead of buying school lunch was availability of beverage vending machines in schools."[2] Changes such as removing sugary beverages (soda, sport drinks), chips, and candy bars from a la carte cafeterias, vending machines, and school stores are essential to improved dietary behavior.[3]

Soft drinks are known to contribute to childhood obesity because of the increased energy intake and the subsequent decline in nutrient intake. There have also been associations made between adolescent soft drink consumption and mental health problems. "High consumption levels of sugar-containing soft drinks were associated with mental health problems among adolescents even after adjustment for possible confounders."[4] The mental health problems examined in this Norwegian study were mental distress, hyperactivity, and conduct problems, whereas the control variables were eating habits and social and behavioral variables.

A healthy diet is crucial to reducing a child's risk of several physical health problems, and recent evidence suggests that good nutrition also protects mental health.[5] The need for schools to prioritize nutrition by fostering a healthy food environment targets the child obesity epidemic, although exercise in schools is another critical part. Students spend a significant amount of their day at school, and therefore to get the recommended amount, exercise must be a fundamental component of their day. The physical activity guidelines for children and adolescents are at least one hour (60 minutes) each day.[6]

A study looking at several health indicators in school-aged children including depression found that greater health benefits were linked to more physical activity. Although vigorous-intensity exercise may provide the greatest health benefits for children, it is indicated that even for those considered high-risk such as the obese, small amounts of physical activity can be beneficial.[7] A variety of physical activity opportunities in schools can be offered to accommodate students of all fitness levels and ages.

Similarly, the National Association of Sport and Physical Education recommends 150 minutes of physical education a week for the entire school year. Middle schools and high schools are encouraged to provide 225 minutes a week throughout the entire school year.[8] Nationally, there are severe shortcomings in physical education recommendations, with only 6.6% of first grade children meeting guidelines.[9] The relationship between physical activity and better health outcomes has been largely demonstrated. School as an institution has a meaningful impact on student lives and can counter the effect of obesity by providing sufficient physical education programs and recess.

The direct association between the lack of physical activity and childhood obesity is well documented.[10] Daily physical activity suggests beneficial health affects according to this study by Katz and colleagues.[10] It is also important to consider the relationship between physical fitness and academic achievement. "Results show statistically significant relationships between fitness and academic achievement . . . . Promoting fitness by increasing opportunities for physical activity during PE [physical education], recess, and out of school time may support academic achievement."[11]

An argument against daily PE in schools is that it takes away from teaching time. The study by Katz and colleagues[10] discusses a school program that provides multiple, brief, structured physical activity breaks throughout the day. The program is led by classroom teachers, does not require a special facility, and does not reduce teaching time. This particular study and program was implemented in an elementary school; however, "the program can easily be incorporated into almost any school routine."[10]

Nutrition, obesity, and exercise as topics to prioritize for the school day will give students the healthy advantage they need to excel academically and in their lives. The trend of increased poor food options in schools as students get older coupled with declining activity levels as students age creates an environment unfit for academic achievement and positive health choices.[10] Schools can counter this effect by reevaluating existing policies, creating new policies, and introducing programs that value nutrition and exercise.

Exercise and the Brain

Prioritizing academic achievement has in some cases culminated in the elimination of school-based exercise and physical education programs, at great if not yet recognized costs. Humans are designed to exercise, and one of the most prominent findings surrounds the overlapping action between antidepressants and exercise. Antidepressants, from tricyclic antidepressants to selective serotonin reuptake inhibitors, have a common action of increasing brain-derived neurotropic factor (BDNF), which increases neuronal growth in hippocampal regions associated with mood improvement. Stress decreases BDNF, and exercise increases BDNF[12,13]; accordingly, exercise remains a vital component of physical and mental health. Exercise exerts an antidepressant effect in those experiencing clinical depression.[14] Sociocultural factors, however, already influence exercise, because girls prefer "physical activity" to "exercise." The latter term has become associated with body size and sometimes eating disorders.[15] The replacement of physical education with additional classroom instruction and increased academic demands on students seems dissonant with these brain findings and seems to come at a price regarding student mental health.[16]

School Start Times

During adolescence, melatonin levels shift to a later peak, at approximately 11 PM. Adolescents further require approximately 9.25 hours of sleep per night, although currently most high school students receive 7.5 hours or less per night. The vast majority of high school students enter school sleep-deprived. Wahlstrom[17] found that when the high school start time was changed in the Minneapolis area schools from 7:15 AM to 8:40 AM, students slept an additional hour, counter to predictions that they would simply stay up later. Students were less likely to be tardy and less likely to fall asleep during classes, and staff reported that students were "calmer" and there were fewer discipline referrals. These findings have been replicated in multiple other districts, and to date no discordant findings have been reported.[18–21] Resistance, however, to changing school start times remains the rule rather than the exception, but it is usually based on bus scheduling or fears that after-school activities such as sports will be compromised if the school day is extended. Whereas no evidence has disputed the benefits to high school students of delaying school start times, most American school districts continue to prioritize other logistics over this developmental finding.

Adolescent Brain Changes

Recent findings reveal that brain architecture changes markedly in adolescence. Adolescents "prune" brain cells, eliminating neurons not required by the environment, making way for increasing connections between those neurons currently most valued in the adolescent's environment. The brain experiences marked reorganization, with decreases in neurons (gray matter) to allow more efficient transmission by increasing white matter.[22] Educationally, this reorganization represents tremendous brain activity, and thus differences in individual attainment of higher order cognitive skills such as the Piagetian "formal operation" abstract reasoning skills. Whereas some students consolidate abstract thinking by approximately age 14, research reveals that this consolidation is usually accomplished much later, with less than 50% of college freshman having attained these formal operations skills when they enter college.[23]

In addition, adolescents preferentially valence emotional content compared with adults. Using magnetic resonance imaging, Yurgulen-Todd[24] found that adolescents processed photographs of facial emotions more through amygdalar regions, whereas when presented with similar photographs, adults relied more on frontal regions. Using a much larger database, Giedd[25] has replicated these findings. The emotional valence ascribed to content by adolescents results in different reactions to similar stimuli presented, including within school settings. Accordingly, students process stimuli differently than adults and ascribe different emotional meanings (eg, seeing anger rather than fear in facial expressions) than adults. Educationally, this is important in at least three ways.

1. Adolescents process information in emotional centers rather than rational centers of the brain, so information presented in class may stimulate emotional reactions in adolescent students beyond what teachers would anticipate. Efforts to address, examine, and respond to these adolescent reactions should similarly be anticipated by teachers as they prepare lessons.
2. Adolescents seek and read emotions in others (perhaps useful as they begin dating) inaccurately. Accurately identifying emotions of others warrants didactic instruction in how to detect emotions by nuances in facial expressions, voice changes/inflections, eye contact, and body posture. Perhaps this identification is not as automatic as has been previously presumed, despite the significance of these increasingly important (in potential mate selection) and complex (with less parental participation) social interactions.
3. Adolescents may "see" anger where fear is present and thus trust their perceptions and deny adult instruction dissonant with their perceptions. Trusting one's perceptions is an important component in developing self-esteem, so teachers

must be sensitive to the responses and resistance of students to invalidation of these perceptions. Concretely, this will require teachers to objectively examine the evidence to show how conclusions are reached about emotions expressed in photographs, literary descriptions, art, and so forth. Moreover, students may not be able to distinguish their own reactions to material from those identified in a character or photographic subject. Therefore, disentangling student projections of their own reactions from what is actually present may need to gently be addressed. This can be done by clarifying first the students' individual reactions to a photo or description and then a having a discussion/examination of the attributes exemplified in the material that reveal that subject's emotions.

PSYCHOLOGICAL ASPECTS OF SCHOOLING

Developing positive mental health concurrent with academic learning has become increasingly important, particularly as rates of mental illness illuminate the impacts of stress despite living in a better and safer world than ever before.

Mindfulness

Mindfulness has become increasingly infused into school settings. Kabat-Zinn[26] describes it as "the awareness that emerges through paying attention on purpose, in the present moment, and non-judgmentally to the unfolding of experience." Mindfulness is not a strategy, tactic, or philosophy (despite being most often ascribed to Buddhism), but rather a way of living in the present.

Although a variety of mindfulness-based approaches have been investigated in adults, data on the utility of these practices in youth are emerging. Some of the types of therapy teaching mindfulness include mindfulness-based stress reduction (MBSR), mindfulness-based cognitive therapy, dialectic behavior therapy (DBT), and acceptance and commitment therapy. Whereas the methods for teaching mindfulness skills vary, all of these therapies focus on developing and practicing mindfulness. At North Shore Medical Center in Salem, Massachusetts, MBSR has been taught to forty 14- to 17-year-old adolescents using the Cool Minds program developed by Florence Melo-Meyer and colleagues at the Center for Mindfulness at University of Massachusetts Medical School. This is an 8-week program composed of 2-hour weekly sessions and home practice. Cool Minds uses body scan, eating meditation, walking meditation, mindful movements (ie, yoga), and sitting meditation. Several of the practices are summarized by the acronym STOP:

S = Stop the same old reaction and pause, being aware something is difficult. What is difficult to be open to? Where can you soften? Can you try less hard? Effortless.

T = Take a breath through your nostrils; exhale (extending the out-breath relative to the in-breath engages the parasympathetic nervous system and can be calming), then inhale (extending the in-breath relative to the out-breath can engage the sympathetic nervous system and can be energizing). Take these breaths for as long as you need to.

O = Observing your thoughts, feelings, and body sensations, what do you notice?

P = Proceed in a direction that is in line with what is important to you, to your intention.

These practices have been well-received and reported by students as helpful physically, emotionally, and behaviorally. Black[27] reviewed the literature on the efficacy and tolerability of mindfulness practices in children and adolescents and concluded that these practices were accepted by subjects and their families and well-tolerated by the participants. Burke concluded that it was too early to make conclusions about the efficacy of these interventions. There are a variety of excellent resources to learn more about mindfulness and its practice. A few of these include the new programs and current offerings at the University of Massachusetts (www.umass-med.edu/cfm) and the NSCH Web site (http://nsmc.partners.org/web/support/pedi-atrics_resource_center).

Emotional Regulation, Conflict Resolution, and Fundamental Cognitive-Behavioral Training

A more didactic program for promoting emotional growth is available at www. schoolpsychiatry.org. A recent program for facilitating social growth has been created (Brain Driver Education), which includes components of Greene's[28] collaborative prob-lem-solving (CPS), Linehan's[29] DBT and Beck's[30] cognitive-behavioral therapy (CBT). Beck's Web site (www.beckinstitute.org/) provides this traditionally psychiatric con-tent in terms more familiar and palatable to educators. The techniques of CPS emphasize minimizing escalations of conflict, in particular, options for teachers to clarify what issues require adherence by students; options for collaborating by providing and investing students in choices that are feasible, doable, and helpful for both parties in a conflict; and teaching students how to consider the point of view of others.[28] DBT techniques seem useful for emotional regulation. These techniques include breathing exercises, noticing how others are reacting to the student, recog-nizing when emotions are too "cold" or "hot" and interfere with effective decision-making, attending to other sensations (touching comfortable fur, listening to calming or distracting music, and so forth), using medication and calming words ("peace" or "love"), channeling energy effectively by moving one's body, deliberately acting in ways opposite the behaviors associated with distressing emotions, and using desired activities to distract from preoccupations of distressing emotions. CBT techniques are effective and essential, because everyone has moments of distress and these techniques allow one to harness painful emotional reactions by relying on the cognitive skills of the frontal lobes. Specifics include evaluating the evidence for painful conclusions ("I'm stupid because I did badly on a math test"), overvalencing negative events and dismissing positive experiences, projecting what this event realistically portends for the future, assessing pros and cons surrounding choices and anticipating consequences, considering how an event fits in the big picture, and using positive self-talk rather than ruminating about negative attributions.

Preparing Students for Happiness

School practices may benefit from consideration of the emerging science about what cultivates happiness. Layard[31] described seven variables associated with happiness in adulthood:

1. Connectedness and the ability to relate effectively to others
2. Resilience and the ability to respond to adversity
3. Community and the ability to contribute and participate with familiar others
4. Sharing and the ability to partner and rely on others
5. Health and the ability to physically take care of oneself
6. Freedom and the ability to exert control over one's life choices
7. Spirituality and the ability to engage with matters larger than oneself.

These variables provide direction for schools as they prepare students for happi-ness in adulthood. Each of these variables can be infused into the school day, both within curricular content and amid student practices. Consideration of how these attributes can best be fostered in diverse school environments with diverse populations would seem among the more important missions of schools addressing students' future needs.

Curriculum (the "what" that is taught at schools, as compared with instruction, the "how" the curriculum is provided) can be provided to address these topics directly as well as embedded within more traditional school subjects. For example, social skills curriculum such as Garcia-Winner's[32] social behavioral mapping can be integrated in diverse classes. To embed teaching of these attributes within existing curricula, content that identifies how individuals in history and literature have responded to adversity both addresses student fears of failing and identifies specific tactics that students can consider to address their own adversities. For example, Admiral Michael Mullen, chairman of the Joint Chiefs of Staff, recently described how he learned more from his failures than his successes.[33]

Schools have long been described as microcosms of the larger societies they serve. To foster happiness, the meta-messages, or daily practices of school, also warrant mindful review. The school is a community, and how students and staff are valued and encouraged to work together versus autonomously is fundamental in shaping how young people perceive community and their roles. Providing experiences that foster cooperation as much as independent learning and rewarding collaboration among students seem much more viable traits for 21st century survival than conquering others or defeating others in the classroom by earning a higher grade. Whereas curricular content addressing health, including at different life stages, may equip students with practices to maintain their physical health, daily exercise may become more pertinent to all students. This equipping could be done by integrating myriad physical activities such as dance and yoga, easily practiced by most individuals, beyond the expensive extracurricular after-school team activities of fixed duration. Perception of freedom and choice within a school and perception that systems are responsive to their needs and aspirations are important for students to invest in a system. Whereas the separation of church and state has altered presentation of traditional spiritual content, much of fundamental practices stretch across religions and remain appropriate, if not invaluable, to all students; for example, practicing being grateful and learning to forgive remain vital skills easily practiced in all schools and useful to seeing beyond oneself.

SOCIAL PRACTICES

Many school practices throughout the school day, although familiar to generations of students, have not proven effective for cultivating 21st century students. Concretely, the impact and proper place of technology have remained complicated for schools, as has how best to configure the school day and year to optimize learning.

Review of School Variables Influencing Academic Achievement

Hattie[34] has provided the most comprehensive metaanalysis to date of the variables that impact student academic achievement. This metaanalysis involved over 52,000 studies and at least 80 million students. Hattie relied on effect sizes to compare these variables. An effect size (ES) of 1.0 indicates an increase in one standard deviation (SD) on the outcome (here improving school achievement). Practically, a 1.0 SD improvement is associated with advancing a student's achievement by 2 to 3 years (instead of the expected 1 year) or improving the rate of learning by 50%, or a correlation between a variable (eg, amount of homework) and achievement of 0.50. In simpler terms, an ES of 1.0 would be easily visible, as is seeing a person 63 inches tall next to a person 72 inches tall; an ES of 0.29 (the influence of homework on achievement) would resemble the difference between seeing a person 71 inches tall

Table 1						
Evaluation of variables that impact student achievement						
Student Achievement Variable	Metaanalyses	Studies (No.)	People (No.)	Effects (No.)	ES	SE
Teacher	29	2052	500,000	5379	.50	.05
Curricula	135	6892	7,000,000	29,476	.45	.07
Teaching	344	24,906	52,000,000	50,953	.43	.07
Student	133	10,735	7,000,000	37,308	.39	.04
Home	31	1998	10,000,000	3968	.35	.06
School	96	4019	4,000,000	13,609	.23	.07

Abbreviations: ES, error size; SE, standard error. (*Data from* Hattie J. Visible learning: a synthesis of over 800 meta-analyses relating to achievement. New York: Routledge; 2009.)

next to a person 72 inches tall, so there is a difference, but not one that would be visible or clearly different than someone receiving versus not receiving an intervention. The variable categories are described in **Table 1**, which shows that teacher characteristics have the greatest effects (0.50) on student achievement, whereas school characteristics have the least impact (0.23). Collectively, these data emphasize that the teacher variables are most important, then curricular programs that afford planful instruction to fit the diverse needs of students, then the school buildings in which students learn,

Hattie examined a large number of individual variables regarding school, student, curriculum, teachers, and home environment to better clarify contributions of diverse variables toward student achievement. **Table 2** shows the effect sizes of selected notable variables Hattie examined and illuminates that certain variables have significant impacts on student achievement. School variables important for student achievement include total school size (600–900 students in the building) more than classroom size. Allowing students to progress at their own rate, providing stable and cohesive classroom management, and mainstreaming students so that they imitate and learn from their peers seem important; conversely, holding students back (retention) does not have supportive evidence, nor does grouping smart students together (tracking).

Student understanding, appraisal, and investment in their own achievement are most important, as well as student advancement toward formal operations/abstract thinking. Cultivating student motivation remains significant, and early intervention program seem effective. Achievement is influenced by configuring learning tasks to increase student confidence, addressing student fears and anxieties about taking tests, and addressing specific fears such as toward math or science.

Ongoing teacher monitoring of what does and does not work with students remains important to optimize instruction. Teacher-student relationships strongly influence student achievement, as does teaching students how to compartmentalize and access problem-solving approaches to various types of problems. Professional development that is ongoing and provided by new voices from outside the building seems to best enhance achievement. Teacher expectations that stretch but do not break (stress) students yield positive outcomes, and avoidance of labeling students but instead focusing on each student's unique progress enhances achievement. Perhaps counterintuitive, teachers' knowledge of their subject content area seems relatively unimportant.

Table 2
Effect sizes of selected school, student, and teacher variables on student achievement

Variable	Definition and Comments	No. of Studies	Effect Size
SCHOOL			
Acceleration	Allowing gifted students to advance with same mental-age peers	37	.88
Classroom Management	Clarity of purpose; high levels of teacher-student cooperation	100	.52
School Size	Smaller student size associated with greater achievement; optimal size 600–900	21	.43
Mainstreaming	Placing special education students in regular classrooms	150	.28
Class Size	Small class size	96	.21
Ability Grouping	Grouping students based on ability; "tracking"	500	.12
Retention	Repeating a school grade over; non-promotion	207	−.16
STUDENT			
Self-Report Grades	Students' estimates of their own performance	209	1.44
Piagetian Level	Higher levels of cognitive functioning (abstract reasoning, etc)	51	1.28
Motivation	Worthwhile goals, get feedback, affirmation, and sense of autonomy over own learning	322	.48
Early Intervention	School interventions with preschool students	1704	.47
Student Self-Concept	Confidence and "can do" tasks; achievement and self-concept each increase the other	324	.43
Reducing Anxiety	Anxiety particularly for tests and math; most significant from third grade forward	121	.40
TEACHER			
Providing Formative Evaluation	Teachers using data to discern what is effective and what is not for their students	30	.80
Teacher-Student Relationships	Teacher and student mutual regard and respect; person-centered teachers achieved more critical and creative thinking by students	229	.72
Meta-Cognitive Strategies	Thinking about thinking; selecting and monitoring approaches to solve problems	63	.69
Professional Development	Extended over years for staff, provided by external experts	537	.62
Teacher *Not* Labeling Students	Labeling seems more effective for funding than for planning instruction or achievement	79	.61
Teacher Expectations	Emphasizing student progress vs perceptions of student abilities	674	.43
Teacher Subject Matter Knowledge	Teacher's knowledge of subject area content	92	.09

Effective teaching was associated with the following: instruction involving testing of hypotheses (1.09), having deeper understanding of teaching and its effects on student learning (1.02), a sense of control (0.90), high levels of passion for teaching and learning (0.90), a deeper understanding of the subject (not just subject knowledge)

(0.87), being adept at improvisation (0.84), a problem-solving disposition toward teaching (0.82), a positive classroom climate that fostered learning (0.67), and having respect for students (0.61).

Hattie further found that a number of variables historically ascribed significance in student achievement may be less important than previously assumed. Shifting students to different school buildings as they change grade level seems unhelpful (−0.34), and retention of students exerted a negative effect on student achievement (−0.16). Television exerted a negative effect (−0.14), consistent with other findings about the lack of benefit of television in students' lives. Various school practices such as open classrooms and grouping students of differing ages had minimal impact, and programs such as whole language and inductive teaching similarly exerted little effect.

Hattie's analysis of effect sizes concluded that students flourished best when

- they received correct feedback (0.43)
- about previous attempts (0.55)
- related to more difficult goals (0.51)
- that did not discourage (0.33)
- or threaten a student's self-esteem (0.47).

SUMMARY

School practices can be improved by attention to emerging findings in child psychiatry and human development. Adolescent sleep changes, brain maturation, and activity and dietary practices all afford opportunities for school development to improve conditions to optimize learning. Although parents are eager for their children to attain academically, most would prioritize their children developing patterns and skills to become happy, productive social members. School-based programs that promote mental health along with academic achievement are far preferable to perpetuating educational practices that are stressful to students and lack empiric support regarding academic achievement and that contribute to vulnerability to mental illness. Evolving brain and child development findings empower mental health clinicians to shape school practices to improve student successes across academic, emotional, and interpersonal spheres and to enhance student mental health functioning throughout their schooling and into adulthood.

REFERENCES

1. US Department of Agriculture. "National School Lunch Program." Food & Nutrition Service home page. Available at: http://www.fns.usda.gov/cnd/lunch. Accessed September 14, 2011.
2. Park S, Sappenfield WM, Huang Y, et al. The impact of the availability of school vending machines on eating behavior during lunch: the Youth Physical Activity and Nutrition Survey. J Am Diet Assoc 2010;110(10):1532–6.
3. Briefel RR, Wilson A, Gleason PM. Consumption of low-nutrient, energy-dense foods and beverages at school, home, and other locations among school lunch participants and nonparticipants. J Am Diet Assoc 2009;109(2 Suppl):S79–90.
4. Lien L, Lien N, Heyerdahl S, et al. Consumption of soft drinks and hyperactivity, mental distress, and conduct problems among adolescents in Oslo, Norway. Am J Public Health 2006;96(10):1815–20.
5. Diet and mental health. Mental health foundation home page. Available at: http://www.mentalhealth.org.uk. Accessed September 14, 2011.

6. Physical activity for everyone: Guidelines: Children | DNPAO | CDC. Centers for disease control and prevention. Available at: http://www.cdc.gov/physicalactivity/everyone/guidelines/children.html. Accessed September 14, 2011.

7. Janssen I, Leblanc AG. Systematic review of the health benefits of physical activity and fitness in school-aged children and youth. Int J Behav Nutr Phys Act 2010;7:40.

8. NASPE physical education guidelines. American alliance for health, physical education, recreation and dance - AAHPERD. Available at: http://www.aahperd.org/naspe/standards/nationalGuidelines/PEguidelines.cfm. Accessed September 14, 2011.

9. Fernandes M, Sturm R. Facility provision in elementary schools: correlates with physical education, recess, and obesity. Prev Med 2010;50(Suppl 1):S30–5.

10. Katz DL, Cushman D, Reynolds J, et al. Putting physical activity where it fits in the school day: preliminary results of the ABC (Activity Bursts in the Classroom) for fitness program. Prev Chronic Dis 2010;7(4):A82.

11. Chomitz VR, Slining MM, McGowan RJ, et al. Is there a relationship between physical fitness and academic achievement? Positive results from public school children in the northeastern United States. J Sch Health 2009;79(1):30–7.

12. Duman RS, Monteggia LM. A neurotrophic model for stress-related mood disorders. Biol Psychiatry 2006;59(12):1116–27.

13. Duman RS. Neurotrophic factors and regulation of mood: role of exercise, diet and metabolism. Neurobiol Aging 2005;26(Suppl 1):88–93.

14. Dunn AL, Trivedi MH, Kampert JB, et al. Exercise treatment for depression: efficacy and dose response. Am J Prev Med 2005;28(1):1–8.

15. Loman DG. Promoting physical activity in teen girls: insight from focus groups. MCN Am J Matern Child Nurs 2008;33(5):294–9 [quiz: 300–1].

16. Biddle SJ, Asare M. Physical activity and mental health in children and adolescents: a review of reviews. Br J Sports Med 2011;45(11):886–95.

17. Wahlstrom K. Changing times: findings from the first longitudinal study of later high school start times. NASSP Bulletin 2002;86(633):3–21.

18. Hansen M, Janssen I, Schiff A, et al. The impact of school daily schedule on adolescent sleep. Pediatrics 2005;115(6):1555–61.

19. Owens JA, Belon K, Moss P. Impact of delaying school start time on adolescent sleep, mood, and behavior. Arch Pediatr Adolesc Med 2010;164(7):608–14.

20. Wahlstrom K. School start time and sleepy teens. Arch Pediatr Adolesc Med 2010;164(7):676–7.

21. Wolfson AR, Carskadon MA. Understanding adolescents' sleep patterns and school performance: a critical appraisal. Sleep Med Rev 2003;7(6):491–506.

22. Giorgio A, Watkins KE, Chadwick M, et al. Longitudinal changes in grey and white matter during adolescence. Neuroimage 2010;49(1):94–103.

23. Lawson AE. Relationships among level of intellectual development, cognitive style, and grades in a college biology course. Science Education 1980;64(1):95–102.

24. Yurgelun-Todd D. Emotional and cognitive changes during adolescence. Curr Opin Neurobiol 2007;17(2):251–7.

25. Giedd JN. The teen brain: insights from neuroimaging. J Adolesc Health 2008;42(4):335–43.

26. Kabat-Zinn J. Coming to our senses: healing ourselves and the world through mindfulness. New York: Hyperion; 2006.

27. Black DS, Milam J, Sussman S. Sitting-meditation interventions among youth: a review of treatment efficacy. Pediatrics 2009;124(3):e532–41.

28. Greene RW. What is collaborative problem solving? Lives in the Balance. Available at: www.livesinthebalance.org/what-is-collaborative-problem-solving-cps. Accessed September 16, 2011.

29. DBT resources: what is DBT? Behavioral Tech, LLC. Available at: http://behavioraltech.org/resources/whatisdbt.cfm. Accessed September 16, 2011.
30. Beck Institute for Cognitive Behavior Therapy. Available at: www.beckinstitute.org/. Accessed September 16, 2011.
31. Layard R. Happiness: lessons from a new science. New York. Penguin; 2005.
32. Garcia-Winner. Social Thinking. Available at: www.socialthinking.com. Accessed September 16, 2011.
33. Military.com. Mike Mullen tells all to Letterman. Under the Radar. Available at: http://undertheradar.military.com/2011/06/mike-mullen-tells-all-to-letterman/. Accessed September 16, 2011.
34. Hattie J. Visible learning: a synthesis of over 800 meta-analyses relating to achievement. New York: Routledge; 2009.

Maximizing the Uptake and Sustainability of School-Based Mental Health Programs: Commercializing Knowledge

Darcy A. Santor, PhD[a], Alexa L. Bagnell, MD, FRCPC[b],*

KEYWORDS
• Mental health • School-based interventions
• Knowledge mobilization

The number of school-based interventions focusing on health and mental health promotion or illness prevention now number well over a thousand.[1] Several critical reviews[2,3] and metaanalyses[4] have been published documenting the clear benefit of such programs for mental well-being, illness prevention, and even academic success, and a number of permanent repositories that rate and list effective school-based programs have been established. (For a review, see Santor and colleagues.[5]) However, the efforts to date in implementing health promotion or illness prevention programs on a mass scale have not succeeded. This lack of success does not diminish the importance of continuing efforts to improve the effectiveness of school-based programs, for which effect sizes can be at times modest, but the scope of child mental health problems and resource limitations highlights the need to now balance program development and improvement with maximizing uptake and implementation. Knowledge mobilization is a much discussed concept in this process, but less has been focused on the role of the clinician in evoking change and new approaches. This article outlines what is known about knowledge exchange and mobilization and introduces a business lens in considering school-based mental health programs uptake and sustainability. The individual clinician can have significant impact in advocacy and ongoing education by promoting strategies that work within a school setting for both patients and the whole school population. In building

---

The authors have nothing to disclose.
[a] School of Psychology, University of Ottawa, Ottawa, ON, Canada
[b] Department of Psychiatry, Dalhousie University, IWK Maritime Psychiatry, 5850/5980 University Avenue, Halifax, NS B3K 6R8, Canada
* Corresponding author.
E-mail address: Alexa.Bagnell@iwk.nshealth.ca

Child Adolesc Psychiatric Clin N Am 21 (2012) 81–92
doi:10.1016/j.chc.2011.09.004   childpsych.theclinics.com
1056-4993/12/$ – see front matter © 2012 Elsevier Inc. All rights reserved.

these relationships, the opportunity now presents for changing how mental health and mental illness are approached and supported in the school setting.

A BRIEF OVERVIEW: WHAT WE KNOW ABOUT FOSTERING UPTAKE AND SUSTAINABILITY

Research and innovation regarding knowledge exchange has been considerable and now pervades most fields in the life sciences. The field has witnessed a growth in terms of new models of knowledge exchange as well as new terminology.[6] This brief overview reviews a few key studies examining the effectiveness of programs designed to change clinical practice and the factors necessary in implementing and sustaining programs. Application of these concepts and strategies to school-based programs in mental health can provide an opportunity for improving uptake and longer term success.

MAXIMIZING UPTAKE

Maximizing the uptake of child and youth mental health programs is about encouraging schools to implement programs designed to promote health, prevent illness, and/or address systemic problems. Despite widespread acknowledgement of the benefits of school-based mental health programs, many schools are still reluctant or reticent about implementing programs for a number of reasons that range from (a) readiness and capacity issues to (b) uncertainty about what type of program should be implemented and how to select a program. In many cases this implementation may mean that a school will need to adopt or change policy or practice, which is analogous to the considerable investments that have been made to change physician practice and implement new guidelines. In the absence of studies directly examining the uptake of school-based programs, the results of studies in other domains may be relevant.

Grol and Grimshaw[7] reviewed some 54 studies examining the effectiveness of interventions designed to change clinical practice among physicians. Conclusions from this systemic review are presented in **Table 1**. Results of this review suggest that person to-person contact in the form of outreach visits or interactions among small groups of people are among the most effective strategies of modifying clinical practice of health professionals. Similar results have been cited alongside other reviews.[2,8–10] Assuming these findings generalize to a school-based setting, this result suggests that the most effective way to encourage schools to adopt school-based programs will be through more interactive, person-to-person, or small group meetings. Strategies such as policy papers or knowledge sharing conferences by themselves will likely be insufficient. A more recent review of the literature undertaken by the Continuing Medical Education (CME) Guidelines Panel reached a similar conclusion[11]:

> Based on the literature, didactic education, including traditional lecture-style teaching, as a single mode of instruction, was found to be the least effective form of learning, in terms of . . . knowledge retention, skill application and patient outcomes . . . . In contrast, the most effective CME incorporates a diversified approach to education, utilizing a combination of multimedia, multiple instructional techniques and multiple exposures to topic areas.

In summary, efforts to foster the uptake of school-based programs will be most effective if they are frequent, sustained, and in person and use multiple approaches to communicate that message. In simpler words, routing a school to a paper that details effective practices will most likely be less effective than having a consultant extrapolate findings to that school with staff who practice and refine their repertoire of skills.

Table 1
Strategies designed to change clinical practice among physicians and conclusions about their effectiveness

Strategy	Conclusion
Educational materials	*Mixed effects*
Conferences	*Mixed effects*
Interactive small-group meetings	*Mostly effective*
Educational outreach visits	*Especially effective*
Use of opinion leaders	*Mixed effects*
Different educational strategies	*Mixed effects*
Feedback on performance	*Mixed effects*
Reminders	*Mostly effective*
Mass media campaigns	*Mostly effective*
Multiprofessional collaboration	*Effective*
Combined interventions	*More effective than single interventions*

Effective strategies are in bold text
Data from Grol R, Grimshaw J. From best evidence to best practice: effective implementation of change in patients' care. Lancet 2003;362:1225–30.

There have been some successes in the education arena. One of the most sustained and successful efforts was led by the Collaborative for Academic, Social, and Emotional Learning (CASEL) group, which has supported and promoted the development, validation, and dissemination of programs that teach social emotional learning. Social emotional learning programs have been widely adopted in some states in the United States and have been shown to be effective not only for improving mental well-being but also academic outcomes.[4,12] Illinois passed legislation in 2004 requiring that "every Illinois school district shall develop a policy for incorporating social and emotional development into the district's educational program." The Academic, Social, and Emotional Learning Act (HR 4223) currently before the US Congress proposes that more resources and emphasis be placed on social emotional learning in the educational system.

MAXIMIZING SUSTAINABILITY

Although the factors that contribute to maximizing uptake may also facilitate the continued and sustained use of a program, the sustainability will depend on a variety of other factors that range from (a) demonstrating ongoing value and relevance to educators and students; (b) minimizing the degree of burden on both users and stakeholders to access, use, and benefit from the program; (c) securing sufficient resources to support ongoing development and revision of materials; and (d) providing timely and relevant effectiveness and outcome data. Each of these factors is essential to ensuring that interest in and use of the resources is sustained. Literature from the field of education has identified necessary components to sustainable programs in the school setting (**Box**1).

Denton and colleagues[13] identified the following factors that seem to influence sustainability of high-quality implementation in reading programs: teachers' acceptance and commitment to the program; presence of a strong school site facilitator to support teachers as they gain proficiency; feelings of professionalism and self-determination among teachers; teachers provided with professional development

---

Box 1
Common components for sustainable school education programs

- The program must be seen as valuable and effective by those within the school.
- There should be local ownership of the program by teachers and administrative staff.
- The program must be well supported by both the participating school and the program developer/coordinator.
- The program must be flexible and adaptable to the needs of the school.

(training, in-class coaching, and prompt feedback); programs are perceived by teachers as practical, useful, and beneficial; administrative support and leadership; and instructional practice valued by the school leaders and administration including long-term support. Elias and colleagues[14] identified the following factors for sustainability in social/emotional learning programs presence of a program coordinator or committee to oversee implementation and resolution difficulties; involvement of individuals with a good moral sense and ownership for the program; ongoing process of formal/informal training; inclusiveness among students; visibility in the school; components that foster mutual respect and support among students; varied and engaging instructional approaches; links to stated goals of schools or districts; and consistent support from school principals.

REFRAMING KNOWLEDGE TRANSFER AND EXCHANGE

Knowledge transfer and exchange (KTE) has been described as an interactive process involving the interchange of knowledge between research users and researcher producers. The impetus for focusing on knowledge transfer, whether in areas of medical knowledge or other program, arose in response to the significant challenges experienced in transferring knowledge from researchers to end users, whether these are practitioners or policy makers. After more than a decade of research into the factors influencing knowledge transfer the challenges remain significant, and it is now clear that the barriers to program uptake will not be solved by understanding the difficulties as a question of knowledge transfer or exchange alone.

In the presidential address at the Canadian Psychological Association in 2010,[15] an international leader in the development of school-based programs targeting bullying behavior reviewed a number of important obstacles to program uptake and implementation. These challenges range from the inadequacy of short-term grants to the new challenges researchers are often required to undertake, namely functioning as advocate, marketer, trainer, quality assurance manager, and continued evaluator of the program. As others have done, this investigator emphasized the ongoing need for further research but also acknowledged that the challenges in advancing mental health promotion and illness prevention will not be solved by research in isolation. The concept of knowledge mobilization incorporates KTE, as well as implementation in the real world.

Since the seminal work of Weiss,[16] knowledge mobilization research has seen the development of an increasing number of models, paradigms, and terminology.[6] The barriers to mobilizing knowledge created by relying on researchers from academic departments to push new knowledge into community and clinical settings where it could appropriately be pulled in and used are considerable.[17,18] These limitations of knowledge mobilization research come from both critical reviews that have directly questioned the generalizability of KTE studies[19] and the firsthand experience of anyone who has worked in implementing and sustaining a program, intervention, or set of guidelines. Knowledge mobilization requires expansion and inclusion of other frameworks such as business models in order to address the full scope of the challenge.

NEW FRONTIERS: COMMERCIAL MODELS OF KNOWLEDGE MOBILIZATION

Health research is seeking new ways to mobilize knowledge. The US-based Center for Advancing Health recently sponsored a conference titled Getting Tools Used, in which they sought to better understand how to increase the uptake of health decision-making tools. Despite the existence of a variety of health decision-making tools from physician and hospital report cards to comparative information guides on the benefits of different treatment and procedures, use of health care decision aids is infrequent despite significant investments.

In a recent Kaiser Family Foundation survey, only 14% of adults indicated they had seen and used comparative health quality information for health insurance plans, hospitals, or doctors in the past year.[20]

By examining the practices of successful companies reviewed in *Consumer Reports, eBay* and *US News & World Report*, the Center for Advancing Health review panel identified six key messages for health care stakeholders regarding the manner in which health decision-making tools should be developed and disseminated:

- Tools must provide information that is otherwise unavailable to the consumer.
- Health care decision support tools must meet a ready audience.
- Tools created within the health care industry will have less resonance with consumers than those created by independent (less biased) groups.
- Tools must have a strong brand identity.
- Sponsors must develop a self-sustaining business model, allowing the sponsor to reinvest in the evolution of the tool toward the consumer.
- The success of a health care decision support tool largely depends on strategic timing.

There are a number of similarities between these recommendations and the recommendations of reviews examining the factors that affect program implementation, such as the importance of identifying the utility or value of the program, as well as the importance of finding a target audience and providing the program with a high degree of visibility. Some recommendations are arguably new in the sense that they have not traditionally been adopted by researchers or academically based program developers, such as the importance of building a brand identity for the program. Merely convincing end users and stakeholders of the magnitude of the mental health problems facing young people will not be sufficient to motivate stakeholders and decision-makers to implement programs unless they understand the value offered by a specific program and how a specific program will address those needs. Achieving this level of awareness requires strategic marketing and business planning, even after the program, tool, or intervention has been validated as working.

Developing a self-sustaining business model for a program provides the sponsor the means to secure the necessary funding to reinvest in the development of the tool or product. In general, funding for school-based program implementation tends to be limited to an extremely circumscribed intervention trial or program. Program funding rarely if ever is designed to foster or support large-scale expansion. In most cases there is dependence on government agency budgeting for a program that, although a priority area, does not receive ongoing funding. In this regard, any amount of success, expansion, or growth can have an adverse effect on the program because of insufficient financial support. Developing a revenue stream that is directly tied to the growth of the program is essential, otherwise the resources needed to support the expansion of the program will not exist and the program will not be sustained.

COMMERCIALIZING KNOWLEDGE

The report from the Center for Advancing Health marks an important development in thinking about knowledge mobilization from a commercial perspective, emphasizing building the market for the product or program and developing the revenue model to support and grow that program. This concept is fundamentally different from the traditional push-pull paradigm of knowledge mobilization research. Business models have capitalized on translating intellectual property into successful companies.

There are some successful commercial examples in the area of child and youth mental health. The Triple P–Positive Parenting Program is one example. It is described as a system of "easy to implement, proven parenting solutions." This system of solutions "helps solve current parenting problems and prevents future problems before they arise." The program has been a remarkable success, having trained over 55,000 practitioners from the fields of health, education, social services, child care, general practice, and telephone counseling. The program has been implemented worldwide in Australia, New Zealand, Singapore, Hong Kong, Canada, United States, England, Scotland, Belgium, The Netherlands, Curacao, Republic of Ireland, Japan, Germany, Switzerland, Sweden, and Iran. Triple P is a business, and the copyright for the program is held by the University of Queensland, licensed and disseminated through a university-affiliated technology transfer company. Royalties from this dissemination activity are paid to the company and distributed to the university, faculty, School of Psychology, and authors according to the University of Queensland's splits policy for intellectual property.[21] Other school-based programs have also succeeded in commercializing their program. The FRIENDS program based in Australia is a universal school-based anxiety prevention/intervention program that uses a successful business model in training-the-trainer workshops and providing easy to use and easy to disseminate materials. The program research has demonstrated effectiveness in the short term and long term for anxiety prevention and early intervention in Australia,[22,23] has shown similar effectiveness in other developed countries,[24,25] and is currently used in schools in nine countries including Canada and the United States.

These two programs are representative of a growing number of efforts to consider more commercial approaches to the dissemination of knowledge. Business applications of knowledge mobilization include knowledge "brokering"[26] and academic detailing,[27–29] knowledge-value chains,[30] and technology development.[31] Most European and North American universities have technology transfer departments that have begun to approach issues of knowledge transfer from a more commercial perspective.[32]

COMMERCIAL MODELS FOR MAXIMIZING GROWTH AND SUSTAINABILITY

In Canada, there has been an opportunity to implement a mental health literacy and help-seeking program on a large scale (www.myhealthmagazine.net). The core elements of the program were initially developed with research and institutional funds and have been validated in a series of studies.[33–36] However, to implement the program on a large scale, there was need of further funding and a significant overhaul to both the program and dissemination strategy. A commercial model was considered in evaluating and consulting with successful sustainable programs. The model offered a new and fundamentally different perspective. The success of other commercial programs in mental health such as Triple P and FRIENDS and the lessons learned

---

Box 2
Seven characteristics of top-performing high-growth companies

1. Breakthrough Value Proposition

2. Exploit a (High)-Growth Market Segment

3. Find a Marquee Customer to Shape the Product

4. Leverage Big Brother Alliances for Expansion

5. Become Master of Exponential Growth

6. Inside-Outside Leadership

7. The Board of Essential Experts

Data from Thomson DG. Blueprint to a billion: 7 essentials to achieve exponential growth. Hoboken (NJ): John Wiley and Sons, Inc.; 2005.

---

from other health product uptake such as health decision aids emphasized the potential that may exist in developing a commercial model.

What Would Knowledge Mobilization Look Like if Knowledge was a Product and We Went about the Business of Knowledge Mobilization as if It were a Business?

Understanding the key characteristics of highly successful organizations such as eBay or the publishers of *Consumer Reports* is now an industry in its own right, particularly with respect to Fortune 500 companies. Companies such as Starbucks, Google, Microsoft, and even Harley-Davidson make billions of dollars each year from products that are in high demand, often using radically different revenue models. The remainder of this article examines a number of characteristics that distinguish highly successful companies from those that are not.[37] The translation of this information into both small-scale and large-scale knowledge mobilization in the school setting is possible and relevant for all those working with schools, from the individual clinician to the developer of a school-based intervention program. Having an overall strategy that governs the development, implementation, and financing of a program or intervention will ultimately determine its uptake, expansion, and long-term success. Seven characteristics of top-performing high-growth companies, as identified through an analysis of high-growth companies[37] are listed in **Box 2** Many of these characteristics such as a strong value proposition, the importance of meeting the needs of the individuals using the product or program, and the integral role of large influential partners, parallel the same factors affecting knowledge mobilization and program implementation in schools.[13,14]

1. The breakthrough value proposition/target your audience

The first characteristic of highly successful companies is that they articulate a breakthrough value proposition. A value proposition is the fundamental benefit that the consumer obtains from doing business with the company and from the products that the company offers. It may be a product or a service, a service that supports the product, or all. A breakthrough value proposition is what will eventually lead to a product's widespread uptake and use. In the case of Triple P, the breakthrough value proposition is the set of training modules and parenting interventions that allow clinicians to learn the intervention and implement it in a beneficial and effective way.

Developing a value proposition is about (a) identifying who the targeted customer is, (b) determining how the product aligns with the needs of the targeted customer, and (c) articulating what benefits are being delivered to those customers. Developing an effective intervention is valuable, but it does not constitute a value proposition. Moreover, whether or not a program represents a breakthrough value proposition will be determined on the basis of what other products are available that can meet or are perceived to meet the needs of the customer. These other products may include competing interventions designed to target similar problematic child behaviors but will also include every other activity that a school may view as relevant, meaningful, or helpful, whether or not that activity is truly effective, let alone empirically valid.

Developing a new intervention may not be sufficient to garner the interest of the end user. By itself it may not represent a breakthrough value proposition. Accordingly, program developers must address the following questions: (a) what segment of the child and youth mental health market are you targeting, (b) is your program targeting a previously ignored problem, (c) is it an improvement on an existing program, and (d) will it change the way in which treatment programs are delivered (eg, online).

2. Finding a (high)-growth market segment/find an unmet need and innovative approach

The second characteristic of highly successful companies is that they target a high-growth market. From this commercial perspective, maximizing uptake will be most readily achieved by developing or marketing programs that appeal to an important, currently unmet need. This targeting requires thinking carefully about what the new opportunities in the area of child and youth mental health are, or at least the new ways in which child and youth mental health programming can be delivered. Treatment for the large numbers of children and youth with mental illness, despite the devastating impact on individual lives, is arguably not a high-growth market. On the contrary, investment in this sector of health care has been essentially stagnant and chronically underfunded. Accordingly, the high-growth opportunity will not likely come from treating young people in the traditional ways (eg, outpatient services and individual clinicians). Innovative and accessible delivery modalities, capacity building, and infrastructure innovations are all potentially high-growth markets in mental health programs.

3. Find a marquee customer to shape the product/have a champion

The third characteristic of highly successful companies is "marquee customers" who help shape and champion the product or program. In the traditional push/pull model in research and KTE, a lack of personnel in this role is one of the shortcomings in promotion of fidelity over flexibility. Identifying the core components of a program but allowing for school input and some flexibility in the shaping of the product is essential in long-term success. Marquee customers help discover and develop unseen value and increase marketing appeal, and they will also be the primary promoters in the expansion of programs.

4. Leverage big brother alliances for expansion/form alliances

The fourth characteristic of highly successful companies is an alliance with a larger, more influential group that can help garner interest in your program and eventually maximize uptake. In school-based programs, "big brother" alliances are usually large in scope, such as national- or state-level organizations, that may represent the interests of teachers, principal, or guidance counselors. In some instances these alliances may even be with companies that are already selling products or programs to schools and will partner in reselling a product or program that they see as complimentary.

5. Become master of (exponential) growth/have a growth plan

The fifth characteristic of highly successful companies is the ability to master growth—high exponential growth. Fostering and managing high levels of growth is about how to maximize program uptake while sustaining the program. It is also about continuously innovating and finding new ways to address issues while growing the product or program. One element of maximizing growth is to find the means through which the ongoing activities of the programs can be financed. Initially, funding for research and development will be adequate when the utilization of the program is small and fixed. However, as the program grows and is used more broadly, this means being able to deliver the product, service, or program as a unit as fast as demand grows, which generates additional revenue that will be needed to sustain and further develop the program.

Not all programs or services lend themselves to this kind of growth. Providing direct counseling to a young person with mental health difficulties will not fit within this kind of growth model, because the product or service in this instance is produced and consumed by one individual. However, developing a training manual or self-directed online training program does lend itself to this type of growth, because the product or service, once built, can be accessed by an exponentially increasing number of people. In some instances, direct one-to-one counseling will be needed and is the most effective way to address an issue. However, at present providing one-to-one counseling to the 1 in 5 young people with mental illness is not feasible and will likely never be feasible. Direct service on this magnitude of scale is not possible, simply because there are not enough resources (eg, trained professionals) to achieve this task. In this manner, addressing the issue of exponential growth is also about building programs that are in a form that can realistically address child and youth mental health difficulties on the magnitude that is required.

A further element to mastering growth involves treating programs and services as units of growth and tying financial support to the growth unit sales of the program. One of the principal shortcomings of many funding programs and agencies is that they provide fixed amounts, as is usually the case with standard research, development, or capacity-building grants, which does not allow for expansion.

6. Inside-outside leadership/involve stakeholders in operations

Inside-outside leadership is about how the organization allocates responsibility for the daily operations of the organization. Typically, it is the researchers who develop the program or intervention and take on multiple roles, with minimal capacity-building or investment in primary school stakeholders. In the early days of a program it is usually the researcher who is advocate, marketer, trainer, quality assurance manager, and continued evaluator of the program, but at some point the responsibility for each of these varied tasks requires different individuals. The sixth characteristic of highly successful companies is that the roles for developing, marketing, and delivering the program are divided and stakeholders are involved in these roles. In school-based programs, investment of key school partners in operations and responsibility for outcome are important for success.

7. The board of essential experts/collaborate with experts

The seventh characteristic of highly successful companies is the presence of essential experts that provide expertise in key areas such as product development, marketing, and product support. In school-based mental health programs there is often knowledge and research in what works in a research-type setting. However, the expertise in mobilizing this knowledge, culturally adapting program components and creating a sustainable program, is lacking. Identifying the areas that are needed to create a successful business model for your program can provide this expertise without program developers trying to learn a whole set of skills de novo.

WILL A COMMERCIAL MODEL WORK IN CHILD AND YOUTH MENTAL HEALTH?

High-growth companies such as Starbucks, Google, and Microsoft are extremely profitable, and in this regard may be deemed inappropriate as models for consideration in implementing a school-based mental health program. Setting aside the issue of revenue generated and how profits are spent, dispersed, or reinvested, all of these companies share one characteristic that is important for proponents of school mental health programming: they have succeeded in establishing a daily presence in our lives by providing products we value via a sustainable business model. Youth mental health is seen as integral and linked to education and long-term functional outcomes of our most valuable resource, our children, and is increasingly prioritized on government agendas and legislation. Implementation and sustainability remain the primary challenges for school-based mental health programs, and successful business models provide a framework to address these issues.

SUMMARY

Despite the existence of well-validated programs and the near universal acknowledgement of their benefit (at least among mental health professionals), maximizing uptake and ensuring the sustainability of school-based mental health programs and interventions remains challenging. Efforts on the part of national educational organizations (eg, CASEL) are both laudable and essential. These organizations' efforts define the marketplace and have supported the development of such programs. The global success of Triple P and FRIENDS provides evidence that business models in mental health program delivery can work. Much has been learned from research on knowledge mobilization and program implementation about the different factors that can facilitate or impede adopting or utilizing a program successfully. However, there is much that can be incorporated from business models in terms of articulating a value proposition within a marketplace; providing the necessary stewardship for developing, promoting, and supporting a program; and developing the financial mechanism to support and grow a program that keeps step with growth. In learning from successful business characteristics, the importance of relationships is clear and resounds with what we know in the health care setting. Clinicians working with a patient in a school have an impact on how mental health and mental illness is looked at and prioritized in that setting. Program researchers involving and collaborating with stakeholders in identifying needs and investing in success of a program will impact the longevity and success of the initiative. Evidence of effectiveness and need in itself is not enough, and the buy-in of the individuals and groups involved in schools and education is essential in any program or intervention's success.

REFERENCES

1. Weisz JR, Sandler IN, Durlak JA, et al. Promoting and protecting youth mental health through evidence-based prevention and treatment. American Psychologist 2005;60:628–48.
2. Kutash K, Duchnowski AJ, Lynn N. School-based mental health: an empirical guide for decision-makers. Tampa (FL): University of South Florida, Louis de la Parte Florida Mental Health Institute, Department of Child and Family Studies; 2006.

3. National Research Council and Institute of Medicine; O'Connell ME, Boat T, Warner KE, editors; Board on Children, Youth, and Families, Division of Behavioral and Social Sciences and Education. Preventing mental, emotional, and behavioral disorders among young people: progress and possibilities. Committee on Prevention of Mental Disorders and Substance Abuse Among Children, Youth and Young Adults: research advances and promising interventions. Washington, DC: The National Academies Press; 2009.

4. Durlak JA, Weissberg RP. The impact of enhancing students' social and emotional learning: a meta-analysis of school-based universal interventions. Child Dev 2011;82:405–32.

5. Santor DA, Short K, Ferguson B. Taking mental health to school. Policy paper. Ottawa, Ontario (Canada): Ontario Centre of Excellence for Child and Youth Mental Health; 2009. Available at http://www.excellenceforchildandyouth.ca/sites/default/files/position_sbmh.pdf.

6. Sudsawad P. Knowledge translation: introduction to models, strategies, and measures. Austin (TX): Southwest Educational Development Laboratory, National Center for the Dissemination of Disability Research; 2007.

7. Grol R, Grimshaw J. From best evidence to best practice: effective implementation of change in patients' care. Lancet 2003;362:1225–30.

8. Barwick MA, Boydell KM, Stasiulis E, et al. Knowledge transfer and evidence-based practice in children's mental health. Toronto: Children's Mental Health Ontario; 2005.

9. Fixsen DL, Naoom SF, Blase KA, et al. Implementation research: a synthesis of the literature [FMHI Publication #231]. Tampa (FL): University of South Florida, Louis de la Parte Florida Mental Health Institute, The National Implementation Research Network; 2005.

10. Payne AA, Gottfredson DC, Gottfredson GD. School predictors of the intensity of implementation of school-based prevention programs: results from a national study. Prev Sci 2006;7:225–37.

11. Moores LK, Dellert E, Baumann MH, et al. Executive summary: effectiveness of continuing medical education: American College of Chest Physicians Evidence-Based Educational Guidelines. Chest 2009;135:1S–4S.

12. Payton J, Weissberg R, Durlak J, et al. The positive impact of social and emotional learning for kindergarten to eighth-grade students: findings from three scientific reviews. Report prepared for the Collaborative for Academic, Social and Emotional Learning (CASEL). Chicago: Collaborative for Academic, Social, and Emotional Learning; 2008.

13. Denton CA, Vaughn S, Fletcher JM. Bringing research-based practice in reading intervention to scale. Learn Disabil Res Prac 2003;18(3):201–11.

14. Elias MJ, Zins JE, Graczyk PA, et al. Implementation, sustainability and scaling up of social-emotional and academic innovations in public schools. School Psych Rev 2003;32:303–19.

15. Leadbeater B. The fickle fates of push and pull in the dissemination of mental health programs for children. Canadian Psychology 2010;51:221–30.

16. Weiss CH. The many meanings of research utilization. Public Admin Rev 1979;39:426–31.

17. Lavis J, Ross S, McLeod C, et al. Measuring the impact of health research. J Health Serv Res Policy 2003;8:165–70.

18. Lomas J. Using 'linkage and exchange' to move research into policy at a Canadian foundation. Health Aff (Millwood) 2000;19:236–40.

19. Mitton C, Aadair CE, McKenzie E, et al. Knowledge transfer and exchange: review and synthesis of the literature. Milbank Q 2007;85:729–68.

20. Kaiser Family Foundation. 2008 Update on consumers' views of patient safety and quality information. http://www.kff.org/kaiserpolls/posr101508pkg.cfm. Published 2008. Accessed October 12, 2011.

21. Mihalopoulos C, Sanders MR, Turner KM, et al. Does the triple P–Positive Parenting Program provide value for money? Aust N Z J Psychiatry 2007;41:244.
22. Lowry-Webster HM, Barrett PM, Dadds MR. A universal prevention trial of anxiety and depressive symptomatology in childhood: preliminary data from an Australian study. Behav Change 2001;18:36–50.
23. Barrett PM, Farrell LJ, Ollendick TH, et al. Long-term outcomes of an Australian universal prevention trial of anxiety and depression symptoms in children and youth: an evaluation of the friends program. J Clin Child Adolesc Psychol 2006; 35(3):403–11.
24. Conradt J, Essau CA (2003, July). Feasibility and efficacy of the FRIENDS program for the prevention of anxiety in children. Presented at the 24th International Conference: Stress and Anxiety Research Society. Lisbon, Spain, July 2003.
25. Stallard P, Simpson N, Anderson S, et al. An evaluation of the FRIENDS programme: a cognitive behavior therapy intervention to promote emotional resilience. Arch Dis Child 2005;90:1016–9.
26. Ziam S, Landry R, Amara N. Knowledge brokers: a winning strategy for improving knowledge transfer and use in the field of health. International Review of Business Research Papers 2009;5:491–505.
27. Midlov P, Bondesson A, Eriksson T, et al. Effects of educational outreach visits on prescribing of benzodiazepines and antipsychotic drugs to elderly patients in primary health care in southern Sweden. Fam Pract 2006;23:60–4.
28. Ilett KF, Johnson S, Greenhill G, et al. Modification of general practitioner prescribing of antibiotics by use of a therapeutics adviser (academic detailer). Br J Clin Pharmacol 2000;49:168–73.
29. Habraken H, Janssens I, Soenen K, et al. Pilot study on the feasibility and acceptability of academic detailing in general practice. Eur J Clin Pharmacol 2003;59:253–60.
30. Landry R, Amara N, Pablos-Mendes A, et al. The knowledge-value chain: a conceptual framework for knowledge translation in health. Bulletin of the World Health Organization 2006;84:597–602.
31. Lane JP, Flagg JL. Translating three states of knowledge–discovery, invention, and innovation. Implement Sci 2010;5:9.
32. Hagen S. From tech transfer to knowledge exchange: European universities in the marketplace. Business, 2005–2008. Portland Press Limited. Published 2008. http://www.portlandpress.com/pp/books/online/univmark/084/0103/0840103.
33. Santor DA, Poulin C, Leblanc J, et al. Adolescent help seeking behavior on the Internet: opportunities for health promotion and early identification of difficulties. J Am Acad Child Adolesc Psychiatry 2007;46:50–9.
34. Santor D, Bagnell A. Enhancing the effectiveness and sustainability of school-based mental health programs: maximizing program participation, knowledge uptake and ongoing evaluation using internet based resources. Advances in School Mental Health Promotion 2008;1:17–28.
35. Santor DA, Kususmakar V, Poulin C, et al. Facilitating help seeking behavior and referrals for mental health difficulties in school aged boys and girls: a school-based intervention. J Youth Adolesc 2006;36:741–52.
36. Santor DA, Poulin C, Leblanc J, et al. Evaluating effectiveness of school based health centers: facilitating the early detection of mental health difficulties. J Adolesc Health 2006;39:729–35.
37. Thomson DG. Blueprint to a billion: 7 essentials to achieve exponential growth. Hoboken (NJ): John Wiley and Sons, Inc.; 2005.

Generalized Anxiety Disorder in the Classroom

Katharina Manassis, MD, FRCPC

KEYWORDS

- Generalized anxiety disorder
- Attention deficit-hyperactivity disorder • Self-efficacy • Student
- Learning disabilities

Generalized anxiety disorder (GAD) in children is characterized by excessive, uncontrollable worries accompanied by 1 or more physical symptoms of anxiety (eg, stomachaches, headaches, or insomnia) and causing impairment in daily functioning.[1] It typically has an early age of onset, chronic course, and high association with other anxiety disorders and depression[2] and affects up to 10% of children and adolescents.[3] These findings suggest that 2 to 3 children in a given classroom will experience significant distress and impairment related to GAD. If one includes children who are distressed but have more limited impairment (so-called *high trait anxiety*), the number affected is even higher.

A large longitudinal study[4] found that self-reported symptoms of anxiety in first-grade children were predictive of adaptive functioning, including educational attainment, in grade 5. This was surprising, as studies of cognitive abilities in anxious children have generally failed to find any deficits relative to nonanxious children,[5] and mild levels of anxiety tend to increase motivation and even enhance cognitive performance.[6] Thus, it appears that these anxious but cognitively intact children are failing to reach their academic potential. In addition, educators often report difficulty managing children's anxiety in the classroom. Because only a minority of anxious children are likely to come to the attention of child psychiatrists and psychologists,[7] there is clearly a role for classroom-based interventions to improve the academic outcomes and overall well-being of these children.

Several programs focused on treating children's anxiety in school settings have been developed and evaluated. Unfortunately, these programs often are costly and require considerable staff training, so it is not feasible to implement them in all educational settings. Moreover, not all anxious children suffer from GAD. Other disorders and certain life circumstances can evoke the same symptoms. Extensive diagnostic testing, however, is also not feasible in most schools. Therefore, this chapter briefly reviews key aspects of assessing children's anxiety in school settings

Department of Psychiatry, University of Toronto, Hospital for Sick Children, 555 University Avenue, Toronto, ON M5G 1X8, Canada
E-mail address: Katharina.manassis@sickkids.ca

Child Adolesc Psychiatric Clin N Am 21 (2012) 93–103
doi:10.1016/j.chc.2011.08.010
1056-4993/12/$ – see front matter © 2012 Elsevier Inc. All rights reserved.

and key findings from evidence-based programs but emphasizes practical strategies that may be helpful for children showing signs of GAD in the classroom.

DOES THIS CHILD HAVE GAD?

As mentioned, excessive worry is the hallmark of GAD, and it is often accompanied by signs of physical tension. In the classroom, however, children do not always volunteer the fact that they are worried. Instead, they show other behaviors that are suggestive of worry. These are listed in **Table 1** and can include perfectionism, being easily overwhelmed by large assignments, excessive concern about tests, preoccupation with time limits, inability to tolerate uncertainty or changes in routine, excessive requests for teacher reassurance, and interpersonal sensitivity (eg, sensitivity to criticism).[8] Students with GAD may exhibit 1 or more of these features.

There are several other reasons why students may exhibit these behaviors. Learning problems and attention deficit-hyperactivity disorder (ADHD) both commonly evoke anxiety symptoms in school settings and should be suspected in students who do not exhibit anxiety symptoms in other settings. For example, adolescents with poor reading skills were found to have high rates of GAD, social anxiety, and functional impairment even when controlling for the presence of ADHD.[9] GAD and ADHD also show a high rate of co-occurrence (up to 20% in some studies),[10] so this possibility should be considered in students who appear anxious and struggle academically. A psycho-educational assessment may be helpful to clarify the cause of anxiety symptoms in students with academic difficulty.

GAD symptoms may also co-occur with other childhood anxiety disorders or with other mental health problems, such as mood disorders or autism spectrum disorders. The co-occurrence of anxiety disorders is common in children,[5] especially among GAD, social phobia, and separation anxiety disorder. These are sometimes difficult to distinguish and often respond to similar interventions. If co-occurring mental health problems include nonanxiety symptoms (eg, social inappropriateness or stereotypies suggesting autism spectrum disorders or persistent low or irritable mood suggesting depression), a detailed diagnostic assessment by a child psychologist or psychiatrist may be indicated.

Psychosocial stresses or medical conditions can also evoke anxiety symptoms in children and adolescents. The latter may include thyroid problems, use of certain medications, or consumption of caffeinated beverages[11] and can be assessed by the child's family doctor or pediatrician. Bullying, abuse, severe family conflict or family separation, or severe student-teacher conflict are common stresses that may result in anxiety symptoms that mimic GAD. Children often are reluctant to discuss these issues with adults, so one should be alert to these possibilities and further investigate (or contact the appropriate authorities in the case of abuse) if they are suspected.

Finally, if one hopes to identify anxious children in a school proactively, there are several teacher rating scales that may be helpful. The long form of the Conners' Teacher Rating Scales Revised includes an anxiety-focused subscale that may be helpful.[12] Recently, the School Anxiety Scale-Teacher Report, a 16-item anxiety-focused instrument, has been validated in children ages 5 to 12 years[13] and was found to discriminate between clinically anxious and nonanxious children with some consistency. It contains a subscale specific to GAD. Anxiety ratings vary a great deal across informants though,[14] so one cannot conclude that a particular child has GAD based on teacher ratings alone without corroborating information from the child and the parents.

Table 1
Manifestations of generalized anxiety and corresponding classroom strategies

Manifestation	Classroom Strategies
Perfectionism	• Normalize mistakes or reframe them as learning opportunities • Encourage rough drafting and brainstorming • Emphasize quantity rather than quality of work • Encourage handing in imperfect work • Do not extend deadlines • Do not draw undue attention to mistakes
Fear of large assignments	• Break the project or large assignment into chunks • Help the student schedule a time to do each chunk • Have the student hand in one chunk at a time and praise each submission • Help the student focus on his or her strengths and the ability to improve performance with effort
Test anxiety	• Take test in a separate, quiet room • Allow extra time to complete test • Avoid unexpected quizzes or tests • Encourage a few slow, deep breaths before starting • Encourage finding one easy question to start with
Anxiety about time pressure	• Avoid "minute math" or other tests with time pressure • Allow extra time to complete tests • Encourage finishing one task at a time versus multitasking • Avoid serious or humiliating penalties for minor tardiness for all students
Intolerance of uncertainty	• Provide clear daily schedules and clear deadlines • Warn the student if something out of the ordinary is planned and help him or her prepare • Use checklists and other visual reminders of tasks and upcoming events • Develop a coping plan for unexpected events
Excessive reassurance seeking	• Answer question and repeat once using the same words (to minimize chances of confusion) • Encourage the student to save further questions for a specific time, and then be available at that time • Positively reinforce gradually increasing amounts of independent work completion • Provide realistic but reassuring information about specific worries or fears • Encourage writing down worries rather than going to an adult right away
Physical signs of anxiety	• Do relaxation exercises with the whole class • Encourage slow, deep breathing when the student appears stressed • Have a quiet place where the student can go for a few minutes if he or she is overwhelmed

(continued on next page)

Table 1 (continued)	
Manifestation	Classroom Strategies
Interpersonal sensitivity	• Maintain a calm, patient tone of voice
	• Avoid penalizing the whole class when a few students misbehave
	• Provide calm but firm limits for misbehavior
	• Set reasonable academic expectations that take anxiety into account but are not too low and do not single out the anxious student
	• Address any teasing or bullying among students
	• Positively reinforce help seeking in those who are afraid to ask for help

EVIDENCE-BASED PROGRAMS

School-based interventions evaluated in children with GAD or anxiety symptoms have been largely cognitive-behavioral in nature. Cognitive-behavioral interventions (CBT) emphasize replacing anxious thoughts with more adaptive thoughts (termed *cognitive restructuring*), relaxation to reduce physical symptoms of anxiety, and encouraging children to face feared situations they may be avoiding. These interventions are not necessarily specific to GAD, as anxiety disorders often co-occur in preadolescent children[5] and often respond to similar interventions. The most widely used is the FRIENDS program for childhood anxiety,[15–18] a universal school-based intervention that has been evaluated in comparison with nonintervention conditions when administered by psychologists, graduate students, school nurses, and teachers. Decreased anxiety symptoms are reported across studies regardless of leader type relative to nonintervention.

Unlike universal programs, which are provided to all students in a given class, indicated programs focus exclusively on students with elevated anxiety symptoms.[19] The Penn Resiliency Program for children and adolescents, for example, uses CBT principles to reduce symptoms of depression as well as anxiety and has included a mix of teachers and graduate students as group leaders.[20,21] Dadds and colleagues[22,23] studied 7 to 14 year olds anxious either by self-report or teacher nomination, randomized to a school-based child- and parent-focused CBT intervention administered by psychology graduate students or a monitoring (nonintervention) group. Both groups improved immediately postintervention, with lower rates of anxiety disorders for the active intervention at 6 months and 2 years but not 1 year. Misfud and Rapee[24] randomized children with anxiety symptoms to either "Cool Kids," an 8-session CBT program provided by mental health professionals, or waitlist control. They found significant group differences in anxiety symptoms at 4 months postintervention. Finally, Manassis and coworkers,[25] randomized children with elevated anxiety symptoms to either school-based CBT or an activity control condition of equal duration and found significant reductions in anxiety symptoms in both groups postintervention and at 1-year follow-up but no between-group differences. Interestingly, high therapist use of positive reinforcement and low amounts of free time during sessions (implying a high degree of structure) were predictive of reductions in anxiety symptoms.

Neil and Christensen[19] reviewed this literature thoroughly and identified 27 school-based CBT trials focused on anxiety at that time. Most reduced symptoms of anxiety in the short term but with a wide range of effect sizes (0.11–1.37), and few included active control conditions or long-term follow-up. Trials with active control conditions typically had smaller effect sizes (ie, smaller differences between intervention and control conditions) than those with nonintervention control conditions.

One of the few non-CBT interventions recently evaluated was termed an *incremental theory of intelligence manipulation*.[26] Twenty-eight adolescents with GAD were randomly assigned to the incremental theory condition or a control condition and administered a coding task. They were told this task measured intelligence, which often is assumed to be an inborn trait. In the incremental theory condition, they were also told that they could improve their performance through effort, and in the control condition they were not. Adolescents in the incremental theory condition performed better on the task and experienced less state anxiety than those in the control condition.

The above findings suggest that children's anxiety symptoms may decrease somewhat in response to different school-based interventions, some of which may be easier to implement than a full CBT program. Providing a high degree of structure, providing frequent positive reinforcement, and expressing confidence that the child can improve academic performance through effort are classroom strategies supported by the literature that many teachers already use. From a cognitive perspective, these strategies may increase the child's sense of self-efficacy and increase the predictability of classroom routines and expectations. These effects are likely to be therapeutic for children with GAD, as they often underestimate their abilities and find uncertainty or unpredictability difficult to tolerate. Recent findings suggest that, in addition to formal CBT, classroom strategies for children with GAD that increase self-efficacy and predictability may be worthwhile.

A PRACTICAL APPROACH TO THE STUDENT WITH GAD

A practical, helpful approach to the student with GAD can include attention to the classroom environment, attention to the environment outside the classroom (ie, school, parents, and professionals working collaboratively on the student's behalf), and specific coping strategies for the anxious student. Each of these aspects will now be discussed.

The Classroom Environment

Helping the child with GAD cope well at school involves attention to the environment around the child as well as specific anxiety-focused strategies. Most anxious children prefer not to be singled out from their peer group, so whenever possible, interventions should either include the whole class or assist the anxious child in unobtrusive ways. Simple relaxation exercises that involve the whole class and systemic interventions to address teasing or bullying are examples of the former approach; providing positive reinforcement for progress with anxiety-related behaviors privately at the end of the school day (rather than announcing it to the class) is an example of the latter approach.

Consistent with the literature, a classroom environment that has predictable schedules and routines is usually experienced as reassuring by the child with GAD. For many anxious children, the need for predictability also includes the need for 1 person (ie, the teacher) to be clearly in charge. Teachers who manage student misbehavior calmly but firmly are often experienced as more reassuring than those who tolerate a somewhat chaotic classroom environment.

Finally, children with GAD sometimes personalize penalties or criticisms directed at the whole class or at other students. It is therefore important that no student's behavior is managed in harsh or humiliating ways, and whole-class penalties should be avoided. For example, I once saw a child who was anxious to the point of daily vomiting before school because his teacher tried to discourage tardiness by forcing late students to wear late-slips pinned to their shirts the whole day.

The Environment Outside the Classroom

Students with GAD usually do best when expectations of them are consistent at home, at school, and among involved professionals. Consistency avoids confusion (which tends to be anxiety provoking) and increases predictability. Therefore, good working relationships between teachers, parents, and professionals should be nurtured.

It may be helpful for the student to have an individualized education plan developed with input from parents, professionals, and the student herself. Input from 1 or more of the student's previous teachers may also be helpful. Academic expectations should take anxiety into account (eg, by reducing time pressure or incorporating other strategies from **Table 1**) but not be too low. Significantly modified academic expectations should only be set for students with GAD if they also suffer from learning disabilities.

In addition to having clear academic expectations, it is often helpful to make a plan for reducing any anxiety-related behaviors that may be interfering with academic performance, such as those listed in the left hand column of **Table 1**. A gradual, patient approach with consistent positive reinforcement for progress is usually most helpful. Parents often know what type of positive reinforcement is likely to motivate their children. For example, some students respond better to verbal praise, others to stickers, others to bonus marks or other academic incentives, and others to more tangible rewards provided at home.

Parents may also benefit from reading books about child or adolescent anxiety such as *Keys to Parenting Your Anxious Child*[27] or *If Your Adolescent Has An Anxiety Disorder*[28] to better support the child with GAD at home. In addition, all adults around the child with GAD can be helpful by modeling calm, effective coping with day to day stresses. Children often emulate these adult behaviors, even if they do not acknowledge or even realize it.

After developing the individualized education plan, 1 or more regular methods of communication between home, school, and professionals are needed. A written agenda to communicate daily concerns and a weekly telephone call or e-mail may be needed, at least initially. If a student is not making progress, it may be helpful to have further parent-teacher meetings, or further professional consultation.

Specific Strategies for Students with GAD

As mentioned, recent findings suggest that promoting students' sense of self-efficacy and creating a predictable environment are helpful to children with GAD. Developing specific strategies based on these general principles, however, requires some thought. To organize this thinking, it is helpful to identify which of the classroom manifestations of GAD listed in **Table 1** are most prominent in a given child. Then, strategies suitable to that manifestation can be developed. The strategies listed in **Table 1** are ones that I have often suggested when consulting to educators about children with GAD, but the list is not exhaustive. There are undoubtedly other ways of helping children with GAD feel safer and more confident in their abilities, and I have often been impressed by the creativity of educators in discovering these.

Perfectionism

Worrying about the consequences of minor mistakes can result in perfectionism in children and adolescents with GAD. Perfectionism can be debilitating because some children with this characteristic are so fearful of doing their school work imperfectly that they do it very slowly, repeatedly erase it, or avoid doing it altogether. Ultimately, these students must recognize that their fear of mistakes is exaggerated and desensitize to it by being allowed to make some mistakes.

Educators can help by normalizing mistakes (eg, saying "Everyone makes mistakes sometimes" or "Oh well . . . nobody's perfect") or reframing mistakes as helpful learning opportunities. When students are producing little work because of perfectionism, it may be helpful to avoid grading work for a period and instead positively reinforce quantity rather than quality of work handed in. Encouraging students to produce rough drafts or to brainstorm ideas about a topic before writing about it can also help those who are paralyzed by perfectionism. Encouraging students to hand in incomplete or obviously imperfect work helps them face their fear of mistakes but is too anxiety-provoking for many students with GAD to tolerate. If the student has some anxiety management strategies or is working with a therapist, however, it may be a useful approach.

Drawing undue attention to mistakes (eg, marking them with a large red "X" or displaying test scores for others to see) can exacerbate perfectionism. Extending deadlines for assignments can also exacerbate perfectionism by allowing students excessive time to review, edit, and hone their work to achieve perfection, rather than facing their fear of imperfection.

Fear of large assignments

Students with GAD often are overwhelmed when facing large assignments. They typically underestimate their own ability to manage a "big project" and overestimate the difficulty of the task. Some may not even look at the task, assuming it is impossible to manage.

"Chunking" is a favorite educational strategy for this problem. The teacher helps the student break a large assignment into smaller chunks and helps him or her make a schedule for tackling each chunk. Then, rather than having a single deadline for the whole project, the teacher asks the student to hand in 1 chunk at a time and provides positive reinforcement for doing so. If the student is still struggling, the size of the chunks can be reduced, or the teacher can ask leading questions to prompt work production. The student can also be reminded of past successes with work completion to increase his or her sense of self-efficacy. Rewarding partial success or evidence of effort (rather than praising only complete pieces of work) can also build confidence, especially if the student is told that performance will improve further with continued effort.

Test anxiety

Students with GAD often worry about the consequences of poor school performance and may exaggerate these. For example, they may assume that 1 bad mark will result in failing a subject or even a whole year. Therefore, indicating clearly how much a particular test or examination is worth in relation to the student's final grade in a subject may alleviate some anxiety. Having tests at predictable times rather than having students do unexpected "pop quizzes" is also typically helpful. Students who are very worried about time pressure may benefit from extra time to complete tests, and those who worry about being distracted by others may benefit from writing tests in separate, quiet rooms.

All students can be encouraged to take a few slow, deep breaths before a test or examination starts and to find at least 1 easy question to do first to build confidence. These strategies often reduce anxiety for everyone.

Anxiety about time pressure

Students with GAD commonly worry that they will not have adequate time to finish academic tasks. Allowing extra time on tests has already been mentioned as a helpful way to reduce this anxiety. Working quickly can still be encouraged if desired, however, by using incentives. For example, a student could be told "When you finish your work, you can get back to reading your favorite book." This approach creates a flexible time limit that reduces anxiety but still motivates the student to work at a reasonable pace.

Multitasking sometimes increases anxiety about time limits, because when the student is working on several tasks concurrently it seems like none are ever finished. Therefore, encouraging students to work on 1 task at a time is often helpful. Tests and tasks that deliberately increase time pressure (eg, "minute math") are generally not helpful, as they increase anxiety and therefore result in an underestimate of the anxious student's true abilities. Because students with GAD tend to react to others' misfortunes as well as their own, punishing minor tardiness severely in any student can increase perceived time pressure for the student with GAD. Rewarding consistent punctuality is usually a less anxiety-provoking method of keeping the class on time.

Intolerance of uncertainty

Difficulty tolerating uncertainty is considered a key feature of GAD,[1] and this may explain why increasing predictability has been found to be so helpful for anxious students. Strategies that create a more predictable classroom environment include having clear daily schedules, having clear deadlines, and using checklists or other visual reminders of upcoming events. The student with GAD may also need warnings about changes in routine or special events such as school field trips.

Particularly challenging situations can include school fire drills and having a substitute teacher, as it is often not possible to anticipate these events. It may be helpful to make a coping plan for the student with GAD to keep at his or her desk in case such an event occurs. The plan may include slow, deep breathing, sitting next to a less anxious "buddy" (who is also aware of the plan), going to the office if very anxious, and (in the case of a substitute teacher) providing a written summary of the student's needs to minimize changes in routines and expectations.

Excessive reassurance seeking

When students are anxious they may seek reassurance repeatedly or in inappropriate ways that are disruptive to the class. For example, the anxious student may continue to ask questions about a topic after the rest of the class has moved on to another. Providing a reassuring answer to a question may prompt several follow-up questions, typically beginning with "But what if . . .?"

It is important for teachers not to become angry or frustrated in response, as emotional reactions typically heighten anxiety. Instead, it is better to respond calmly with a simple explanation, and repeat it once if needed using exactly the same words so as to minimize the chances of confusion. If excessive reassurance seeking is chronic, other helpful strategies may include encouraging the student to save further questions for a specific time, positively reinforcing gradually increasing amounts of independent work completion, or encouraging the student to write down worries rather than going to an adult right away.

If a student is participating in a therapy focused on recognizing anxiety and coping with it (eg, cognitive behavioral therapy), he or she may eventually be able to practice self-reassurance when prompted to do so by an adult. For example, the adult could say "You seem anxious about this issue. What could you do to handle that anxiety?" or "What could you say to yourself to reduce the anxiety?" Encourage parents to seek such therapy for their children if the children often struggle with anxiety-related behaviors in class.

Physical signs of anxiety

Physical signs of tension or anxiety such as headaches, stomachaches, frequent urination, or hyperventilation can all be manifestations of GAD. Students who experience them should be encouraged to take a few slow, deep breaths, and may need to have a quiet place to retreat to such as the school office or the library. In the case of urinary frequency, having a bathroom signal that the student can use to excuse themselves unobtrusively is often helpful, although many of these students can increase the time between bathroom visits with practice. Students should never be barred from the bathroom if distressed, however. Regardless of the symptom, students usually do best if encouraged to return to class within a few minutes. Calling home or asking to be picked up from school should be discouraged unless there are definite signs that the student is physically ill (for example, fever or vomiting).

All students can benefit from learning how to do simple relaxation techniques, such as slow, deep breathing or progressive muscle relaxation. Devoting a health class to relaxation at least once a year is often beneficial to all.

Interpersonal sensitivity

Anxious students sometimes report that teachers yell at them, although, in truth, the teacher is speaking sternly but not raising his or her voice. This occurs because students with GAD are sometimes exquisitely sensitive to signs of interpersonal conflict or disharmony.

To a degree, anxious students must desensitize to these signs, but teachers who often speak harshly can still be difficult for these students to tolerate and can distract them from academic work. Beyond maintaining a calm tone of voice, other helpful strategies can include not penalizing the whole class for a few students' misbehavior (anxious students may take whole-class penalties personally), providing calm but firm limits for misbehavior of any student (having the teacher clearly in charge often reduces student anxiety), and addressing any teasing or bullying among students (reducing the chances of the anxious student being victimized; also see section on the classroom environment above). Some students with GAD also avoid asking for help when needed, because they fear teacher criticism in response. For these students, help seeking may need to be deliberately encouraged.

SUMMARY

Interventions for students with GAD require attention to contextual factors both within and outside the classroom. They often are based on the principles of increasing environmental predictability and increasing the student's sense of self-efficacy. Good judgment is sometimes needed to determine which strategies constitute reasonable accommodations to the student's anxiety and which constitute an excessive deviation from usual school expectations. The latter can single out students unnecessarily or limit their academic progress. Working closely with parents and mental health professionals involved in the student's care is most likely to ensure a consistently helpful approach.

REFERENCES

1. American Psychiatric Association. Diagnostic and statistical manual of mental disorders, 4th edition. Washington, DC: American Psychiatric Association, 2000.
2. Kessler RC, Keller MB, Wittchen HU. The epidemiology of generalized anxiety disorder. Psychiatr Clin North Am 2001;24:19–39.
3. Keeton CP, Kolos AC, Walkup JT. Pediatric generalized anxiety disorder: epidemiology, diagnosis, and management. Paediatr Drugs 2009;11:171–83.
4. Ialongo N, Edelsohn G, Werthamer-Larsson L, et al. The significance of self-reported anxious symptoms in first grade children: prediction to anxious symptoms and adaptive functioning in fifth grade. J Child Psychol Psychiatry 1995;36:427–37.
5. Canadian Psychiatric Association. Anxiety treatment guidelines initiative. Clinical practice guidelines: management of anxiety disorders (special populations: children). Can J Psychiatry 2006;51(Suppl 2):1S–92S.
6. Petri HL. Motivation: theory, research, and applications, 3rd ed. Belmont, CA: Wadsworth Publishing Company; 1991.
7. Offord D, Boyle M, Racine Y. Canada Child Health Survey: Children at risk. Toronto, Ontario: Queen's Printer; 1989.
8. Giordano G. Rechanneling anxieties. In: Walz GR, Bleuer JC (eds). Helping students cope with fears and crises. Ann Arbor, MI: ERIC Clearinghouse on Counseling and Personnel Services; 1992.
9. Goldston DB, Walsh A, Mayfield Arnold E, et al. Reading problems, psychiatric disorders, and functional impairment from mid- to late adolescence. J Am Acad Child Adolesc Psychiatry 2007;46:25–32.
10. Manassis K. When ADHD co-occurs with anxiety disorders: effects on treatment. Expert Rev Neurother 2007;7:981–8.
11. Manassis K. An approach to intervention with childhood anxiety disorders. Can Fam Physician 2004;50:379–84.
12. Conners CK. Conners' Teacher Rating Scales Revised 2011. Available at: http://psychcorp.pearsonassessments.com. Accessed September 29, 2011.
13. Lyneham HJ, Street AK, Abbott MJ, et al. Psychometric properties of the School Anxiety Scale—Teacher Report (SAS-TR). J Anxiety Disord 2008;22:292–300.
14. Barbosa J, Manassis K, Tannock R. Measuring anxiety: parent-child reporting differences in clinical samples. Depress Anxiety 2002;15:61–5.
15. Barrett PM, Lock S, Farrell LJ. Developmental differences in universal preventive intervention for child anxiety. Clin Child Psychol Psychiatry 2005;10:539–55.
16. Bernstein GA, Layne AE, Egan EA, et al. School-based interventions for anxious children. J Am Acad Child Adolesc Psychiatry 2005;44:1118–27.
17. Lock S, Barrett PM. A longitudinal study of developmental differences in universal preventive intervention for child anxiety. Behav Change 2003;20:183–99.
18. Stallard P, Simpson N, Anderson S, et al. The FRIENDS emotional health programme: initial findings from a school-based project. Child Adolesc Ment Health 2007;12:32–7.
19. Neil AL, Christensen H. Efficacy and effectiveness of school-based prevention and early intervention programs for anxiety. Clin Psychol Rev 2009;29:208–15.
20. Gilham JE, Reivich KJ, Freres DK, et al. School-based prevention of depression and anxiety symptoms in early adolescence: a pilot of a parent intervention component. School Psychol Quart 2006;21:323–48.
21. Gilham JE, Reivich KJ, Freres DR, et al. School-based prevention of depressive symptoms: a randomized controlled study of the effectiveness and specificity of the Penn Resiliency Program. J Consult Clin Psychol 2007;75:9–19.

22. Dadds MR, Spence SH, Holland DE, et al. Prevention and early intervention for anxiety disorders: a controlled trial. J Consult Clin Psychol 1997;65:627–35.
23. Dadds MR, Holland DE, Spence SH, et al. Early intervention and prevention of anxiety disorders in children: Results at 2-year follow-up. J Consult Clin Psychol 1999;67:627–35.
24. Misfud C, Rapee RM. Early intervention for childhood anxiety in a school setting: outcomes for an economically disadvantaged population. J Am Acad Child Adolesc Psychiatry 2005;44:996–1004.
25. Manassis K, Wilansky-Traynor P, Farzan N, et al. The Feelings Club: a randomized controlled trial of school-based intervention for anxious and depressed children. Depress Anxiety 2010;27:945–52.
26. Da Fonseca D, Cury F, Fakra E, et al. Implicit theories of intelligence and IQ test performance in adolescents with Generalized Anxiety Disorder. Behav Res Ther 2008;46:529–36.
27. Manassis K. Keys to parenting your anxious child. 2nd edition. Hauppauge, NY: Barron's Educational Series, Inc; 2007.
28. Foa EB, Wasmer-Andrews L. If your adolescent has an anxiety disorder. New York: Oxford University Press; 2006.

Treating Adolescents with Social Anxiety Disorder in Schools

Julie L. Ryan, PhD[a], Carrie Masia Warner, PhD[b,c,d],*

KEYWORDS

- Social anxiety • Adolescents • School-based treatment
- Dissemination

Social anxiety disorder, characterized by significant discomfort and avoidance of social or performance situations,[1] is among the most common mental disorders in children and adolescents. Recent estimates indicate that 6% of children[2,3] and 12.1% of adolescents meet criteria for this diagnosis.[4] Social anxiety disorder starts as early as age 5 and peaks around age 12.[5] When untreated, it runs a chronic course into adolescence and eventually adulthood.[6,7]

The high prevalence and chronicity is particularly concerning, given the significant disability associated with social anxiety disorder. The clinical picture often involves fewer friends, difficulty participating in classroom activities (eg, answering questions in class, working in groups), and avoiding social interactions (eg, initiating conversations, joining school clubs or sports).[8–10] This social impairment is associated with loneliness, dysphoric mood,[11] and long-term functional impairment, such as difficult life stage transitions, underemployment, suicidal ideation, and risk for substance abuse and depression.[12–20]

Despite its negative impact, the majority of adolescents with social anxiety disorder are likely to remain untreated.[4,12,19,21,22] Recent data estimate that less than 20% of adolescents with anxiety disorders receive treatment,[4] and fewer than 20% of those who do seek services receive interventions supported by

This work was supported by a NIMH grant awarded to Dr Masia Warner, Grant No. R01MH081881.

The authors have nothing to disclose.

[a] School of Psychology, Fairleigh Dickinson University, 1000 River Road, T-WH1-01, Teaneck, New Jersey, USA

[b] Anita Saltz Institute for Anxiety and Mood Disorders, NYU Child Study Center, 215 Lexington Ave, 13th floor, New York, NY 10016, USA

[c] New York University Langone Medical Center, 215 Lexington Ave, 13th floor, New York, NY 10016, USA

[d] Nathan Kline Institute for Psychiatric Research, Orangeburg, New York, USA

* Corresponding author.

E-mail address: carrie.masia@nyumc.org

Child Adolesc Psychiatric Clin N Am 21 (2012) 105–118

doi:10.1016/j.chc.2011.08.011

scientific evidence.[23,24] In contrast to behavior disorders, difficulties may be less apparent to teachers and parents because these children are less disruptive. Many parents do not recognize the extent of their child's impairment[21] or believe that social anxiety is a stage that they will "grow out" of naturally.[25] Because of the nature of the disorder, socially anxious adolescents may not seek help because of potential stigma associated with mental health issues and fear of negative evaluation. Delivering interventions in schools may address the barriers facing youth in need of treatment.

ADVANTAGES OF SCHOOL-BASED TREATMENT

Schools can play an important role in addressing the unmet mental health needs of youth by potentially increasing access to care in a cost-effective manner. This venue provides unparalleled access to youth[26,27] and exemplifies a single setting through which the majority of children can be reached.[28] Social anxiety disorder is particularly suited to being treated in the school setting. First, because of the social nature of the disorder, group treatment may be ideal. Group treatment is logistically challenging in a clinical setting because of variability in diagnoses and scheduling among clients, whereas schools contain many socially anxious students needing intervention. Second, despite the high prevalence[29,19] and impairment associated with social anxiety disorder, these adolescents are rarely identified[21] and, therefore, unlikely to receive help.[12,4,19] Involving schools in the mental health needs of their students creates opportunities to increase identification and treatment of social anxiety disorder by educating teachers and parents about its symptoms and providing support for making appropriate treatment referrals. Finally, intervention implemented within the school setting allows for a real-world treatment approach. That is, the school environment provides opportunities for real-life exposures to commonly avoided situations (eg, answering questions in class, eating in the cafeteria, speaking with teachers, initiating conversations with unfamiliar peers) and for practicing skills in realistic contexts. In addition, peers and teachers with whom socially anxious students routinely associate can be enlisted to support students' progress. When delivering treatment in a natural setting, it is expected that treatment gains may be enhanced and are more likely to generalize to other situations and environments.

Based on these potential advantages, Masia Warner and colleagues[30] sought to develop a treatment program that would draw from empirically supported techniques and could be feasibly implemented in schools. The school-based program, *Skills for Social and Academic Success* (SASS),[30] was derived from *Social Effectiveness Therapy for Children* (SET-C),[31] an empirically supported, clinic-based treatment that consists of 12 individual sessions of behavioral exposures, 12 group sessions of social skills training, and unstructured peer generalization exercises in which socially anxious children practice socializing with nonanxious peers. The emphasis of SET-C on using peers to assist with generalization fits well with the natural availability of same-age peers in the school environment. Clinical trials have demonstrated the efficacy of SASS for adolescents compared with a waiting list[32] and even a credible attention control.[22]

TREATING SOCIAL ANXIETY IN THE SCHOOL SETTING
Overview of Skills for Academic and Social Success

The SASS intervention consists of 12 weekly in-school group sessions (40 minutes) (**Table 1**), 2 group follow-up sessions to address relapse and remaining obstacles, and 2 brief individual student meetings (20 minutes). Additionally, 4 weekend social events (90 minutes; eg, bowling, rollerblading) that include pro-social peers (called

Session	Group
Table 1	
Skills for academic and social success session components	
1	Learning About Social Anxiety
	• Introductions, treatment structure, confidentiality and goals
	• Psychoeducation about social anxiety (e.g., 3-component model)
2	Realistic Thinking
	• Connection between thoughts, feelings, and behaviors
	• Practice challenging negative and unhelpful thoughts
3	Social Skill 1: Initiating Conversations
	• Model friendly and open nonverbal behaviors
	• Practice initiating conversations and provide feedback on nonverbal behaviors
4	Facing Your Fears 1: Rationale and Fear Ladder
	• Present the rationale for exposure exercises
	• Help adolescents construct graduated fear hierarchies
5	Social Skill 2: Maintaining Conversations and Establishing Friendships
	• Learn how to keep a conversation going (eg, when to change topics)
	• Practice maintaining conversations and extend an invitation; provide feedback.
6	Facing Your Fears 2: Conduct Exposures as a Group
	• Practice commonly feared situations (eg, make telephone calls, sing aloud)
7	Social Skill 3: Listening and Remembering
	• Explain how anxiety interferes with being able to effectively listen
	• Practice listening and remembering using characters and personal information
8	Facing Your Fears 3: Conduct Exposures
	• Practice commonly feared situations (eg, start conversations in cafeteria)
9	Social Skill 4: Assertiveness Training
	• Discuss how to refuse requests and practice
	• Learn assertive expression of feelings and needs; practice using "I statements"
10	Facing Your Fears 4: Conduct Exposures
	• Practice exposures higher on the fear ladder and target core fears
11	Facing Your Fears 5: Conduct Exposures
	• Continue practicing exposures higher on the fear ladder
12	Review and Maintenance of Gains
	• Review components of program through individual presentations
	• Explain setbacks and relapse; devise a relapse prevention plan

"peer assistants") are included to provide real-world exposures and skills generalization. Parents are encouraged to attend 2 group meetings (45 minutes) during which they receive psychoeducation regarding social anxiety and learn techniques to manage their child's anxiety and facilitate participation in social activities. Meetings can also be provided for teachers, in which they learn about social anxiety and the program and receive instruction to help students practice classroom exposures. The program is designed to be flexible to accommodate school calendars (eg, vacations and exams) and typically spans about 3 months.

Core Therapeutic Components

SASS treatment groups are small (3 to 6 students), because of time constraints of school class periods, and can be facilitated by 1 or 2 group leaders. The group sessions cover 5 components: (1) psychoeducation, (2) realistic thinking, (3) social skills training, (4) exposure, and (5) relapse prevention.

Psychoeducation

Group leaders provide psychoeducation during the first group session, normalizing the experience of anxiety while presenting a description of the cognitive, physiologic, and behavioral symptoms of social anxiety. Students are encouraged to identify their own anxiety symptoms (ie, feelings of discomfort, worries or "stress") surrounding various social situations and to consider how their social anxiety is maintained through the interaction of negative thoughts, physical sensations, and escape or avoidance. Another goal of session 1 is to introduce motivation for treatment by having each student privately identify which things they would like to change and situations in which they would like to feel more comfortable. Students, as might be expected, are typically reserved and participate minimally at the first group meeting; therefore, the most important goal of the first meeting is to make students feel comfortable.

Session 1 tips for success. To enhance the students' comfort at the initial group session, we recommend that the group leader introduce the group members to one another and avoid placing any students "on the spot." Keeping the atmosphere light, remembering that students may have different areas of social difficulty, and using the word "uncomfortable" rather than "anxious," are some effective strategies to ease students into the first session and encourage their return for session 2.

Realistic thinking

Group leaders focus on cognitive strategies during the second group session. The cognitive strategies, termed *realistic thinking*, were primarily adapted from Ronald Rapee's book. (1998), Overcoming Shyness and Social Phobia: A Step-by-Step Guide.[33] Group leaders highlight the relationship between thoughts, feelings, and behaviors. They then explain that adolescents with social anxiety tend to overestimate the likelihood of the occurrence of negative outcomes and exaggerate the conse-quences of those outcomes if and when they occur. For example, a socially anxious adolescent is likely to assume that, if he extends an invitation to an acquaintance, the acquaintance will reject him or think he is bold and presumptuous for asking, possibly because they are not close friends or for assuming he is worthy of his friendship. Students are taught to identify such negative expectations as unrealistic and to use specific questions to evaluate them more realistically (eg, "Am I exaggerating?" "How many times has this happened in the past?" "Am I being fair to myself?"). Although this is the only group session focused entirely on identifying and challenging negative thinking, these strategies are practiced as needed, which typically occurs during each group and individual session.

Realistic thinking tips for success. The main recommendation for this group is to ensure balance between verbal and active teaching. It is important to provide enough time to practice challenging negative thoughts in role-play scenarios (eg, "You're walking down the hall at school and you see a friend walking toward you. As you pass, you say hello, but she says nothing back."), rather than relying on didactics to illustrate the concept to students. Typically, it is helpful to acknowledge that group members believe their unrealistic thoughts are absolutely true, because they are long-standing patterns of thinking. Therefore, the group members are asked to trust the group leader's past experience with similar students and suspend their doubt and judgment to try these realistic thinking strategies before deciding whether they are helpful.

Social skills training

Improving social skills is helpful for many adolescents with social anxiety, as the development of key social behaviors has often been hindered by inadequate socialization experiences. The 4 social skills sessions include: (1) initiating conversations, (2) maintaining conversations and establishing friendships, (3) listening and remembering, and (4) assertiveness. For each skill, group leaders briefly introduce the concept and rationale and then facilitate group practice through role plays. The leaders choose situations relevant to adolescent experiences (eg, being paired with another student to work on a project or meeting new people through friends) and have the group members practice the skills repeatedly to learn the skill and habituate to the typically ensuing anxiety and awkwardness. Each student participates in at least 2 role plays at each session.

Initiating conversations focuses on the simple ways to begin conversations (eg, commenting on something around you or on something you have in common) and nonverbal communication skills. The second skill session, Maintaining Conversations and Establishing Friendships, focuses on topic transitions and extending an invitation. Socially anxious adolescents often become uncomfortable during conversations and sometimes change the topic of conversation prematurely, making conversations abrupt and awkward. Therefore, during conversational skill practice role plays, students are encouraged to remain on a topic until the group leader gives permission to switch topics. The third skill session involves listening and remembering, and its focus is conquering anxiety interference, which is the tendency to become preoccupied with feelings of anxiety or negative self-evaluations rather than attending to the person speaking. In this session, group members play a memory game in which they disclose social information about themselves to the group, and the group members try to recall that information. During this practice, it is typical for group members to make social mistakes and need to ask one another question to remember the information. Although they make many social mistakes, most group members anecdotally report enjoying the game and becoming more aware of anxiety interfering with their concentration. Finally, the fourth skill session focuses on assertiveness, which includes practice refusing requests and expressing feelings through the use of "I" statements (eg, "I feel frustrated when you borrow my clothes without asking me first").

For all skill practice, both group leaders and members provide feedback by praising positive aspects of role-play performance and by providing suggestions for improvement, such as speaking in a louder voice or increasing eye contact. Specifically, socially anxious adolescents often look unfriendly or unapproachable because of unintended nonverbal behaviors, such as frowning or avoiding eye contact. To address this, all skills groups emphasize teaching students to become aware of these nonverbal messages to others and to reinforce more "friendly" and confident behaviors (ie, smiling, eye contact, speech volume, intonation, and relaxed and engaged body posture). Taking into account the specific needs of each group member and tailoring the skills training to meet the specific needs of socially anxious adolescents is intended to enhance the value of these sessions.

Social skills tips for success. We offer the following strategies to help promote successful skill acquisition. First, group members who struggle with a specific skill may require initial accommodations to be successful (eg, shorter role plays, pairing with more skilled group member, having group members call out alternative sugges- tions, or proving ideas for what to say during the role play). In addition, group members less skilled at giving others feedback may benefit from the overt modeling of appropriate and sensitive feedback to minimize offending fellow students and maintaining group cohesion. During skills training, socially anxious individuals can often become dependent on certain types of conversational questions or statements. Some common examples include commenting on the weather, complimenting the other person, or complaining. Therefore, it is important to train flexibility across skills by having group members generate different dialogues to the same role-play scenarios and brainstorm all the different ways a conversation could be started. Important for all skills taught is repeated practice. Thus, allow time for each group member to role play each skill at least twice in the session, and don't let discussion or questions (eg, the rationale for the exercises) function as avoidance and prevent the full practice of the skills; when time is short, condense explanations and spend time on the practice of skills. Label group members' behaviors as a form of avoidance, when appropriate. Finally, use humor, warmth, and empathy to keep the atmosphere light and pleasant.

Facing your fear

SASS includes 5 exposure sessions, referred to as *Facing Your Fear* sessions, which alternate with the social skill sessions. Group leaders present the rationale and procedure for exposure while emphasizing the role of avoidance in maintaining anxiety and the expectation that anxiety will diminish with increased exposure. Students develop a fear hierarchy, or "fear ladder," that rank orders 10 anxiety-provoking situations, beginning with the least-feared situation. In composing hierar- chies, it is particularly important to tap into the "core fears" surrounding embarrass- ment, rejection, and negative evaluation (eg, "I'm a loser"). Common items that target these specific concerns include giving the wrong answer in class, inviting peers to get together, and making social mistakes, such as forgetting a person's name, tripping in front of a group, arriving late to class, and going to class with messy hair.

During exposure sessions, students practice entering into anxiety-provoking situ- ations while in the group (eg, giving a presentation) or around the school (eg, surveying students in the library). Students are asked to provide subjective units of distress (SUDS) ratings from 1 to 100 (1 = completely calm, 100 = absolutely terrified), before engaging in the exposure, when the exposure has ended, and, ideally, during the exposure. SUDS ratings are expected to decrease by at least 50% by the end of the exposure. If a student is reluctant to engage in the proposed exposure, negative thoughts about the student's expectations are explored briefly, and the feared outcome is compared with the actual outcome after exposure. After exposure exercises, students discuss their experience, and the group provides feedback. Students are given practice exposures between sessions, which are reviewed at the beginning of each session (see Practice Exercises).

Conducting exposure at school provides a meaningful opportunity to capitalize on the school environment by creating a realistic context for encouraging new and challenging behaviors. Being in the school context, we can tailor exposure situations based on the student's difficulties at school (eg, meeting with a teacher for clarification of academic material, approaching a peer in the library or cafeteria) as well as those outside of school (eg, calling a prospective job to inquire about the status of one's application). Exposures implemented during sessions involve other group members, and, because group participants are also school peers, relationships beyond the group may be easily facilitated. Exposure sessions also utilize various school locations. Some common exposures include sending students to the cafeteria to initiate conversations with peers or to purchase and return food, asking questions to the librarian, or visiting the main office to speak to administrative staff. Student pairs might be sent to various locations and return to group to discuss their experiences.

Treatment groups conducted in school also provide the therapist the opportunity to enlist the assistance of school personnel. Because many students experience anxiety talking to authority figures, some exposures might involve interaction with administrators. For example, students may schedule meetings to converse or to make suggestions or complaints. Group leaders facilitate this process by asking school administrators (eg, principal, dean, assistant principal) to be available for these meetings. In addition, group members might deliver the morning school announcements, join a club with another group member, or seek assistance from a teacher who the student finds particularly difficult. Teachers may participate in classroom exposures involving students arriving unprepared or late to class or being reprimanded in front of others, and by assigning leadership roles in group activities. Finally, group members might approach club advisors and coaches to discuss joining clubs or teams.

Adolescents with social anxiety are often hesitant to engage in exposures with a higher potential for negative evaluation or rejection (eg, inviting a peer to get together, attending a party or dance). Unlike traditional clinical settings, integrating treatment into school allows for social risk taking in a more controlled environment. Group leaders and supportive peers are present in the natural setting to encourage and assist students to overcome the anticipatory anxiety involved in attempting more challenging behaviors. This enhances the likelihood that the adolescent carries out the initial attempt at a particularly challenging situation, which increases the chance that the attempt is successful, thus, reinforcing future independent action. For example, group leaders might encourage a student to invite a school peer to get together, knowing that the peer will likely accept their invitation. Exposures conducted in this way optimize the utility of the school environment.

Facing your fears hierarchy building tips for success. When constructing the fear hierarchies, we have found several strategies to be helpful. First, if students have difficulty identifying social situations that make them nervous, ask about situations that they usually avoid, as often they will not consider these situations to be anxiety provoking. Also, group leaders should assist students in identifying specific contexts that make a situation on their hierarchy more or less difficult. For example, if a student is nervous initiating conversations, the group leader should determine whether speaking to someone more familiar or less familiar (eg, friend vs acquaintance) or older or younger (eg, adult vs peer) makes the student more or less comfortable. For a performance situation, the group leader should determine if a familiar versus unfamiliar, or a small versus large audience, is more or less difficult. The situations should then be placed on the hierarchy, with the least distressing variation placed lowest and practiced first. Finally, the first exposure should be constructed to ensure that the student is capable of handling it with minimal difficulty and that it will be a successful and positive experience.

Facing your fears practice tips for success. When helping students practice exposure situations on their fear hierarchies, it is valuable to keep in mind that students may not be accurate in the fear ratings they assign to each situation because of lack of experience with the feared scenario. Therefore, when conducting exposures, it is important to monitor the student's level of distress and, if the exposure is much more difficult than expected (eg, appears to be an "8 out of 10" even though the student had initially rated it lower), modify the task to make the experience more manageable. This strategy can also be helpful when an adolescent is extremely resistant to the initially proposed exposure. More specifically, briefly explore the cognitions that may be contributing to the hesitation and, if the reluctance persists, propose a similar exposure that the adolescent finds less daunting. For example, if a student is resistant to the idea of approaching an unfamiliar peer in the cafeteria to start a conversation, a more structured version of this exposure, such as asking the unfamiliar peer survey questions as a mock class assignment, may be an acceptable alternative. Finally, be aware of excessive time spent engaging in cognitive restructuring or discussions about the usefulness of a proposed exposure (eg, "But I'll never need to ask the librarian for assistance"), because these discussions may function as avoidance, squandering time needed for exposure practice.

Practice exercises

Each group session ends with the assignment of practice exercises. These exercises are designed to help students apply the skills they have learned in group to situations that occur between group sessions. Practice exercises, such as practicing realistic thinking, starting conversations, refusing requests for favors, and performing a step on the fear ladder, are critical for extending skills practiced in group to additional situations inside and outside of school and fostering a structure for long-term success. Although formal worksheets are provided, typically students do not complete these, and it appears sufficient to have students report specific recollections of skill use during the prior week. The group leader asks the group member what they were expecting to happen before engaging in the practice and what they experienced during and after engaging in the practice. This level of review appears to increase accountability for completing practice exercises between sessions; however, for group members who consistently fail to practice skills between sessions, the group leader should use the individual meeting to help the student problem solve any obstacles to practice. Being in the school environment lends additional benefits, as group leaders can provide additional support to students' between-session practice by eliciting the assistance of school personnel, such as informing a teacher that the group member will be asking for clarification of academic material, or having a pro-social peer remind the group member that their club meets today.

Relapse prevention

The final group focuses on maintenance of gains and relapse prevention. During the final group session, each member gives a speech about their experience in the program focusing on what they have learned and accomplished and areas for continued improvement. After the presentations, group leaders discuss how to maintain gains and goals for continuing progress and how to manage inevitable setbacks to avoid relapse. Group members outline the warning signs of emerging symptoms and strategies for reversing them. We have found that it is important to highlight the inevitability of setbacks while instilling confidence in the students' capability to handle the situations as they were able during the group.

Individual Sessions

Students attend one or two 15-minute individual sessions to discuss treatment goals, complete fear hierarchies, and address any issues that may be interfering with progress that they are not comfortable discussing during the groups. In addition, these meetings may be used for customized cognitive restructuring, review of social skills that are particularly challenging, individual exposures (eg, calling to invite someone to get together), or additional exposures that the student has been avoiding. These meetings provide opportunities to strengthen rapport between the student and group leader and to identify potential stressors other than social anxiety (eg, being bullied, academic difficulties, parental divorce) that may be impacting group participation or their ability to practice outside of session.

Follow-up Sessions

Group follow-up or booster sessions are conducted monthly for 1 or 2 months after termination. The intention of these sessions is to monitor progress, problem-solve obstacles to continued improvement, and encourage and sustain practice. Additional exposures may be performed during group booster sessions.

Social Events

Three to 4 weekend social events are considered helpful for skill generalization and practice. The events, such as bowling, miniature golf, rollerblading, and laser tag, are attended by group leaders, group members, and peer assistants from the students' high schools (see later discussion). The activities provide group members the opportunity to practice social skills and allow for exposure to several commonly avoided situations (eg, attending a social event without friends or with unfamiliar peers, initiating conversations, performing in front of others), while providing group leaders with a sample of the students' functioning in social situations. Group leaders actively facilitate the first event and encourage interaction between group members and peer assistants; however, at later events, group leaders limit their presence facilitating to only when a group member is having particular difficulty.

Social events tips for success. When planning the first social event, we recommend picking a more structured activity (eg, bowling), because they tend to be less intimidating and provide more support for group members who may be less practiced in certain social skills. As the group progresses, later social events should be less structured (eg, going to a restaurant, having a board game party) to challenge the group members to use their skills. Exposures can be built into every kind of social event. For example, group leaders may encourage group members to order the food at the event, offer food or drinks to others, divide up players to make teams, and approach unfamiliar peers. Finally, picking a venue that is less public or scheduling the event during a time that classmates not involved in the group will be less likely to be present may increase participation by group members who are sometimes concerned about confidentiality. Alternately, to make students more comfortable and address confidentiality concerns when outside of school, it might be helpful to give the group a club name (eg, Peer Leadership Club) and consider the group leader accompanying the students to be the club's advisor.

Peer Assistants

Peer assistants are helpful, friendly, and pro-social students identified by school personnel to assist with the SASS program. After the first year of the program, peer assistants are ideally students who have previously completed the SASS program. The primary role of peer assistants is to create a positive experience for group members at social events. Peer assistants bring enthusiasm and energy to the events and ensure that all students are integrated in the group activities. Peer assistants may also facilitate peer support within the school environment through assisting with exposures and skill practice, such as bringing a group member to join a school club or having conversations in the cafeteria or hallways.

Selecting peer assistants tips for success. We recommend briefly interviewing each student who is identified as a potential peer assistant. During the interview, we suggest asking about their involvement in extracurricular activities, how the student responds to bullying, and what they would do if they noticed a shy student sitting by themselves during an activity. In our experience, the best peer assistants are not necessarily the most extroverted students but rather are students who are caring and empathic.

Parent Meetings

Two parent meetings are conducted during the intervention. These meetings are essential because many parents have a limited understanding of the symptoms and impairment associated with social anxiety. Parents often are frustrated and over-whelmed by their children's avoidance behaviors (eg, refusing to order food in restaurants) and fail to understand the extent of their suffering. Therefore, the first meeting provides psychoeducation about social anxiety, whereas the second meeting addresses skills being taught in the SASS program and how parents can support their children's skill use. Psychoeducation helps parents better understand their children's experiences and the anxiety underlying avoidance behavior. Parental behavior is also discussed in a nonjudgmental way (eg, it is natural for parents to remove their children from distressing situations or to assist them when they are struggling), as it plays a role in the development and maintenance of anxiety. The first parent session concludes by explaining the SASS program structure and rationale.

During the second parent meeting, common parental reactions to children's anxiety are reviewed. Throughout the second parent meeting, unhelpful and helpful ways to react to children's anxiety are contrasted. Through a facilitated discussion, parents are encouraged to allow for increased autonomy (which leads to more effective coping and problem-solving skills) and discontinue providing excessive reassurance, being overly directive, and allowing avoidance of social interactions. Parents are instead instructed to encourage positive coping, prevent avoidance, and communicate empathy. Helping children feel more confident and competent is vital for nurturing a successful transition into young adulthood.

Parent meetings tips for success. The main recommendation for conducting the parent meeting is to be empathic and supportive to parents regarding 2 common extremes, either desiring to protect their child and allowing their child to avoid distressing situations or alternatively becoming frustrated and being too direct and harsh when pushing their child. We suggest validating the parents' attempts to be helpful and focus on more effective strategies to prevent avoidance without being overly directive. For instance, rather than providing their children scripts of what to say or structuring their children's social plans, parents may prevent avoidance more successfully by offering to provide transportation to an event or encouraging contact with friends. Often parents do not realize the messages their protective behaviors are sending to their child (eg, the world is a scary place or you can't handle this without my help). Being compassionate and validating regarding parents' unhelpful behaviors is the key to a successful parent meeting.

Involvement of Teachers

Another benefit to school-based intervention involves educating teachers about social anxiety and obtaining their collaboration to assist shy students. Group leaders can meet with 2 or 3 of a student's teachers and their school counselor to educate them about social anxiety and the rationale for exposure exercises. Teachers often are aware of students who have difficulties participating in class or giving oral presentations and are glad to be involved. The group leader can ask teachers to collaborate on appropriate and graded exposures (eg, answering questions in class) and to continue communication with the clinician conveniently through e-mail or by phone to provide updates and feedback regarding the student's progress. For instance, if a student fears answering questions in class, the teacher may initially provide the student with the answer to a question before class, followed by providing the student with the question but not the answer, until eventually the student practices answering questions more spontaneously. Teachers can provide feedback about students' progress and identify additional areas to be targeted.

SASS with the Individual

Although SASS was designed to be implemented as a group treatment, there are many strategies that a school counselor or a practitioner in the community can utilize with individual clients within the school environment. The ultimate goal of treatment is to change the adolescent's unrealistic thoughts and avoidance and escape behaviors and to encourage socialization and instill confidence. Most of the session content described can be modified and adapted for an individual in the school environment. For example, exposures can be planned individually with the help of the school counselor or another school contact throughout various settings in school. Some examples of individual exposures include (1) meeting with the principal to discuss the formation of a new club, (2) approaching another student in the library to ask a question, (3) emailing a teacher to set up a meeting time, and (4) texting an acquaintance to make plans for the weekend. Should more support be necessary, the school counselor might enlist the support of a pro-social peer to assist with the student's exposures or for assistance in bringing the student to extracurricular activities. The school counselor is likely aware of a few pro-social peers in the student's school that would embrace the opportunity to encourage a shy student to become more involved in school and social activities. Teachers, once educated by the school counselor, could also assist students with gradual exposures as described previously. Thus, should a group not be feasible, many of the strategies described could be flexibly executed with some minor adjustments.

Feasibility

A fundamental aspect of the SASS treatment program, whether conducted as proposed in a 12-session group format or adapted for individual students, is to involve school personnel. Essential to conducting a school-based intervention is support from the school environment. To successfully conduct the SASS program, it is important to gain the support of school leadership (eg, superintendent, principal, director of guidance) and school personnel (eg, school counselors and teachers) as well as to understand the organizational structure of the school. When working with an individual student, the challenges to engage school personnel are on a smaller scale but may involve more initiative and energy from the individual counselor. School counselors who have previously conducted the SASS program have recommended having 2 counselors act as coleaders, enabling shared responsibility of program implementation (eg, alternate leading groups and attending social events).

Future Directions

Clinical trials have found that SASS is markedly efficacious when delivered by doctoral-level clinical psychologists,[34] even when compared with an attention control condition.[22] For SASS to be accessible to socially anxious adolescents on a larger scale, front-line school practitioners are the logical interventionists. Therefore, a next step toward dissemination and sustainability is to determine if school counselors can implement SASS effectively. Currently, we are conducting a federally funded investigation to evaluate the clinical utility of SASS when delivered by school counselors. Also important will be studies on the type and level of training needed for school personnel with limited or no background in cognitive behavioral therapies (CBT) and ways to maintain treatment fidelity in school settings without the involvement of specialized cognitive behavioral therapy psychologists. This knowledge would inform the dissemination and sustainability of SASS in community contexts as well as cognitive-behavioral interventions for other childhood conditions.

Implications for Practitioners

Based on our experience working with schools, we have found that educating school personnel and parents about social anxiety, including the warning signs (eg, asking to be excused from a class presentation, avoiding school events or parties) and the long-term consequences of untreated social anxiety, may increase recognition of socially anxious adolescents who can sometimes be overlooked. Clinicians should impart to parents, teachers, and school counselors, who may wish to "protect" students from anxiety, that escape and avoidance of anxiety-provoking situations may result in increased anxiety and avoidance. The priority for practitioners is to engage school contacts, such as school counselors, to assist in social skills practice and gradual exposures in the classroom and the social milieu. Allowing socially anxious youth to practice in the natural environment enhances the effectiveness of the skills (eg, realistic thinking, initiating conversations) and the key to the skills being taught in treatment.

REFERENCES

1. American Psychiatric Association. Diagnostic and statistical manual of mental disorders, 4th edition. Washington, DC: American Psychiatric Association; 2000.
2. Chavira DA, Stein MB, Bailey K, et al. Child anxiety in primary care: prevalent but untreated. Depress Anxiety 2004;20(4):155–64.
3. Ruscio AM, Brown TA, Chiu WT, et al. Social fears and social anxiety in the USA: results from the National Comorbidity Survey Replication. Psychological Medicine 2008;38:15–28.
4. Merikangas KR, He J, Burstein M, et al. Service utilization for lifetime mental disorders in U.S. adolescents: results of the National Comorbidity Survey-Adolescent Supplement (NCS-A). J Am Acad Child Adolesc Psychiatry 2011;50:32–45.
5. Kessler RC, Burglund P, Demler O, et al. Lifetime prevalence and age-of-onset distributions of DSM-IV Disorders in the National Comorbidity Survey Replication. Arch Gen Psychiatry 2005;62(6):593–605.
6. Yonkers KA, Dyck IR, Keller MB. An eight year longitudinal comparison of clinical course and characteristics of social anxiety among men and women. Psychiatr Serv 2001;52(5):637–43.

7. Yonkers KA, Bruce SE, Dyck IR, et al. Chronicity, relapse, and illness— course of panic disorder, social anxiety, and generalized anxiety disorder: Findings in men and women from 8 years of follow-up. Depress Anxiety 2003;17(3):173–9.

8. Beidel DC, Turner SM, Morris TL. A new instrument to assess childhood social anxiety and phobia: The Social Anxiety and Anxiety Inventory of Childhood. Psychol Assess 1995;7(1):73–9.

9. Beidel DC, Turner SM, Morris TL. Psychopathology of childhood social anxiety. J Am Acad Child Adolesc Psychiatry 1999;38:643–50.

10. Connolly SD, Bernstein GA, The Work Group on Quality Issues. Practice parameter for the assessment and treatment of children and adolescents with anxiety disorders. J Am Acad Child Adolesc Psychiatry 2007;46(2):267–83.

11. Beidel DC, Turner SM, Young BJ, et al. Psychopathology of adolescent social anxiety. J Psychopathol Behav Assess 2007;29(1):47–54.

12. Essau CA, Conradt J, Petermann F. Frequency and comorbidity of social phobia and social fears in adolescents. Behav Res Ther 1999;37:831–43.

13. Kessler RC. The impairments caused by social phobia in the general population: implications for intervention. Acta Psychiatr Scand 2003;108(Suppl 417):19–27.

14. Liebowitz MR, Gorman JM, Fyer AJ, et al. Social phobia: review of a neglected anxiety disorder. Arch Gen Psychiatry 1985;42(7):729–36.

15. Olfson M, Guardino M, Struening E, et al. Barriers to the treatment of social anxiety. Am J Psychiatry 2000;157:521–7.

16. Schneier FR, Johnson J, Hornig CD, et al. Social phobia: comorbidity and morbidity in an epidemiologic sample. Arch Gen Psychiatry 1992;49(4):282–8.

17. Stein MB, Stein DJ. Social anxiety disorder. Lancet 2008;371(9618):1115–25.

18. Turner SM, Beidel DC, Dancu CV, et al. Psychopathology of social phobia and comparison to avoidant personality disorder. J Abnormal Psychol 1986;95(4):389–94.

19. Wittchen HS, Stein MB, Kessler RC. Social fears and social phobia in a community sample of adolescents and young adults: prevalence, risk factors, and co-morbidity. Psychol Med 1999;29(2):309–23.

20. Woodward LJ, Furgusson DM. Life course outcomes of young people with anxiety disorders in adolescence. J Am Acad Child Adolesc Psychiatry 2001;40(9):1086–93.

21. Kashdan TB, Herbert JD. Social anxiety disorder in childhood and adolescence: current status and future directions. Clin Child Fam Psychol Rev 2001;4:37–61.

22. Masia Warner C, Fisher PH, Shrout PE, et al. Treating adolescents with social anxiety disorder in school: an attention control trial. J Child Psychol Psychiatry 2007;48:676–86.

23. Collins KA, Westra HA, Dozois DJ, et al. Gaps in accessing treatment for anxiety and depression: challenges for the delivery of care. Clin Psychol Rev 2004;24:583–616.

24. Labellarte MJ, Ginsburg GS, Walkup JT, et al. The treatment of anxiety disorders in children and adolescents. Journal of the Society of Biological Psychology 1999;46:1567–78.

25. Masia CL, Klein RG, Storch EA, et al. School-based behavioral treatment for social anxiety disorder in adolescents: results of a pilot study. J Am Acad Child Adolesc Psychiatry 2001;40(7):780–6.

26. Adelman HS, Taylor L. Mental health in schools and system restructuring. Clin Psychol Rev 1999;19:137–63.

27. Weis MD. Expanded school mental health services: A national movement in progress. In: Ollendick TH, Prinz RJ (editors). Advances in clinical child psychology. Vol. 19. New York: Plenum Press; 1997. p. 319–52.

28. Anglin TMMental health in schools: Programs of the federal government. In: Weist MD, Evans SW, Lever NA (editors). Handbook of school mental health: advancing practice and research New York: Kluwer Academic/Plenum Publishers; 2003. p. 89–106.

29. Verhulst FC, van der Ende J, Ferdinand RF, et al. The prevalence of DSM-III-R diagnoses in a national sample of Dutch adolescents. Arch Gen Psychiatry 1997;54: 329–36.

30. Masia CL, Beide, DC, Albano AM, et al. Skills for academic and social success. Available from Carrie Masia Warner C, PhD, New York University School of Medicine, Child Study Center, 215 Lexington Avenue, 13th floor, New York 10016. 1999.

31. Beidel DC, Turner SM, Morris TL. Social effectiveness therapy for children: A treatment manual. Charleston, South Carolina: Medical University of South Carolina; 1998.

32. Fisher PH, Masia Warner C, Klein RG. Skills for social and academic success: a school-based intervention for social anxiety disorder in adolescents. Clin Child Fam Psychol Rev 2004;7:241–9.

33. Rapee's R. Overcoming shyness and social phobia: a step-by-step guide. New Jersey: Jason Aronson Inc; 1998. p. 120.

34. Masia Warner C, Klein RG, Dent HC, et al. School-based intervention for adolescents with social anxiety disorder: results of a controlled study. J Abnormal Child Psychol 2005;33:707–22.

Responding to Students with Posttraumatic Stress Disorder in Schools

Sheryl Kataoka, MD, MSHS[a],*, Audra K. Langley, PhD[b],
Marleen Wong, PhD[c], Shilpa Baweja, MS[d],
Bradley D. Stein, MD, PhD[e,f]

KEYWORDS
- Posttraumatic stress disorder • Psychological first aid
- Trauma • Treatment • Parents • Clinical strategy

The prevalence of trauma exposure among youth is a major public health concern,[1] with a third of adolescents nationally reporting that they have been in a physical fight in the past 12 months and 9% having been threatened or injured with a weapon on school property.[2] Studies have documented the broad range of negative sequelae of trauma exposure for youth, including posttraumatic stress disorder (PTSD), other anxiety problems, depressive symptoms, and dissociation.[3–6] In addition, decreased IQ and reading ability, lower grade point average, more days of school absence, and decreased rates of high school graduation have been associated with exposure to traumatic events.[7,8] Evidence suggests that youth exposed to trauma have decreased social competence and increased rates of peer rejection.[9] Therefore, students who have experienced a traumatic event are at increased risk for academic, social, and

This work was supported by SAMHSA SM59285 (Wong), NIMH 1R21MH082712-01 (Kataoka) and P30MH082760 (Wells).

The authors have nothing to disclose.

[a] Department of Psychiatry and Biobehavioral Sciences, Center for Health Services and Society, Semel Institute, University of California, Los Angeles, 10920 Wilshire Boulevard, Los Angeles, CA 90024, USA

[b] Department of Psychiatry and Biobehavioral Sciences, University of California, Los Angeles, Semel Institute, 300 UCLA Medical Plaza, Suite 1315, Los Angeles, CA 90095, USA

[c] University of Southern California, School of Social Work, 669 West 34th Street, Los Angeles, CA 90089, USA

[d] Department of Psychiatry and Biobehavioral Sciences, University of California, Los Angeles, Semel Institute, Health Services Research Center, 10920 Wilshire Boulevard, Suite 300, Los Angeles, CA 90024, USA

[e] RAND Corporation, 4570 Fifth Avenue, Suite 600, Pittsburgh, PA 15213, USA

[f] University of Pittsburgh School of Medicine, Pittsburgh, PA, USA

* Corresponding author. University of California, Los Angeles, Semel Institute, Center for Health Services and Society, 10920 Wilshire Boulevard, Suite 300, Los Angeles, CA 90024.

E-mail address: Skataoka@ucla.edu

emotional problems as a result of these experiences. School can be an ideal setting for mental health professionals to intervene with traumatized students by supporting both their trauma-related psychological problems and their ability to learn in the classroom. The President's New Freedom Commission Report on Mental Health also highlights the need to improve access to services that address trauma-related mental health problems, especially in naturalistic settings such as schools where youth can readily receive these services.[10]

Types of Traumatic Events that Affect Students

Students can experience a wide range of traumatic events that impact their functioning in school. Some trauma affects students more individually, such as assault, a serious accident, abuse, or community or domestic violence. Other traumatic events impact the entire school community such as a school shooting, terrorist attack, natural disaster, or other incident on campus. Differences in the type of traumatic experience may also influence whether the approach is a school-wide intervention, an individual or group treatment, or treatment targeted to certain school staff or students, each of which is discussed in more detail later in this article. Understanding the types and extent of traumatic events students have experienced, as well as which events are perceived by the student to be the most salient, can be a critical first step in the treatment process.

Posttraumatic Stress Disorder

Although students may experience significant traumatic events, not all develop PTSD. For some, brief distress without significant impairment in functioning may be characterized as a normal reaction. For others, trauma-related symptoms occur in the immediate period following a traumatic event, and if symptoms similar to PTSD are present within the first month following the trauma along with significant distress or impairment, a diagnosis of acute stress disorder may be warranted.

It is estimated that approximately 4% to 6% of youth in the general population nationwide meet criteria for a diagnosis of PTSD following a traumatic event, including symptoms such as poor concentration and intrusive thoughts, which can also severely interfere with school functioning.[2–6,11,12] Since 1987, the childhood manifestations of PTSD symptoms have been described in the Diagnostic and Statistical Manual of Mental Disorders (DSM) and have included specific characteristics that can be seen in children. Further refinement of the PTSD diagnostic criteria are being discussed for the fifth edition of DSM, such as developmental manifestations of PTSD.[13,14] Currently, for a diagnosis of PTSD, the student must experience a traumatic event in which he or she perceives a threat to either self or others and must experience distress (horror, fear, helplessness).[15] For children, this distress can manifest in disorganized behavior or agitation. The three symptom clusters for PTSD include reexperiencing (for children, this can be repetitive play or reenacting the trauma in play), numbing and avoidance (such as avoiding traumatic reminders and talking about trauma, not participating in activities previously enjoyed), and hyperarousal (such as irritability, anger, difficulty sleeping).

Following exposure to a traumatic event, some students may be more likely than others to develop PTSD. Risk factors for PTSD include characteristics of the trauma exposure (greater trauma severity, proximity to the event), individual factors (female gender, history of psychopathologic condition), and parent characteristics (parental psychopathologic condition including PTSD and other trauma-related symptoms, lack of parental support following the trauma). Those students who have had multiple traumatic events and those who experience interpersonal trauma such as an assault can also be at increased risk for developing PTSD.[3–6,11,12,16]

Of those with PTSD, 75% have additional mental health problems such as other anxiety disorders,[6,17,18] depressive symptoms,[4,5,19,20] dissociation,[8] substance use,[21] and aggressive and delinquent behavior.[3,5,22–26] Students exposed to violence may become violent themselves.[27–30]

EVIDENCE-BASED TREATMENTS FOR STUDENTS WITH PTSD

The most often studied treatments for PTSD in youth have been cognitive-behavioral therapy (CBT) approaches. Studies have documented that CBT effectively treats PTSD due to child sexual abuse,[31] intimate partner violence,[32] single-incident trauma,[33,34] comorbid PTSD and substance abuse,[35] and more general community violence.[36–38] According to the practice parameters outlined by the American Academy of Child and Adolescent Psychiatry,[39] when treating PTSD in children, the interventions should include core components of CBT including direct exploration of the trauma, stress management techniques, and correction of cognitive distortions. Treatment should also include collateral sessions with parents for optimal treatment outcomes.[39] One intervention that has been identified as potentially harmful is holding therapy, which forcibly restricts children who have experienced severe and chronic trauma.

Psychopharmacologic treatments have been understudied. A recent review by Strawn and colleagues[40] concluded that pharmacologic agents should not be used as first line treatment for PTSD in youth. Selective serotonin reuptake inhibitors may be helpful, although a recent randomized controlled trial found no difference compared with placebo.[41] Only open trials currently exist for other medications such as antiadrenergic agents, antipsychotic medications, and mood stabilizers.

School-based services may be particularly important for underserved ethnic minority youth who traditionally are less likely to receive such services. For example, a randomized study comparing two efficacious treatments for youth with posttraumatic stress symptoms in post-Katrina New Orleans found that 91% of the youth completed the school-based intervention compared with only 15% who completed the clinic-based intervention.[42]

The Cognitive Behavioral Intervention for Trauma in Schools (CBITS) program, a brief, 10-session group school-based program, has been studied in a quasiexperimental trial (Kataoka and colleagues[36]) and randomized controlled trial (Stein and colleagues[38]), both delivered by school-based clinicians. Findings have demonstrated improvements in PTSD and depressive symptoms among elementary school and middle school students exposed to violence who have received CBITS compared with those on a waiting list.[36,38] Preliminary findings also suggest that this program may have effects on school performance, with students who received CBITS early in the school year doing better in math and language arts than students who received the intervention later that same academic year.[43] The CBITS program was developed in collaboration and partnership with school and community leaders and was specifically designed for school-based delivery for greater fit and sustainability within the school environment. Support for Students Exposed to Trauma (SSET), is an adaptation of CBITS that can be delivered by nonmental–health trained school staff (teachers, school counselors).[44] Results of a small randomized controlled trial suggest that SSET can be delivered by school staff effectively, resulting in modest improvements in trauma-related mental health symptoms. Given the lack of mental health resources typically found in schools and the tremendous need for access to trauma interventions, SSET is a promising early intervention that can be feasibly delivered in schools.

Other trauma interventions have also been developed and studied in the context of schools. The Multimodality Trauma Treatment (MMTT), or Trauma-Focused Coping, is a 14-session group intervention program that adapts basic cognitive-behavioral techniques for students who have experienced a single-incident trauma. Grounded in social learning theory, MMTT uses peer modeling of effective coping, storybooks, narrative exposure, and cognitive games to alleviate trauma resulting from natural disaster, exposure to violence, murder, suicide, fire, or accident. The program is not suitable for children with chronic abuse–related PTSD because the school-based protocol does not incorporate family sessions necessary to address interpersonal victimization.[34] Controlled studies conducted in elementary, middle, and high school demonstrate a marked reduction in PTSD, depression, anxiety, and anger symptoms following the treatment intervention.[33,34]

The University of California Trauma Grief Component Treatment program is designed for adolescents exposed to multiple types of violence and traumatic loss.[45] This intervention includes an extensive assessment protocol followed by 16 to 20 group psychotherapy sessions to mitigate functional impairment associated with PTSD, depression, and grief reactions. Results of a randomized controlled trial conducted with adolescents in postwar Bosnia indicate notable improvement in PTSD, depression, and complicated grief symptoms.[46] Another promising intervention implemented with war-exposed children in Israel is Stress-Inoculation Training. This school-based universal prevention program aims to prevent PTSD by teaching adaptive coping skills and fostering resilience. The curriculum is integrated into mainstream classrooms and teacher-implemented. In a school-matched controlled study, results indicated lower levels of symptoms of posttraumatic stress, depression, and anxiety in those who received the intervention compared with those on a waiting list.[47]

PRACTICAL APPROACHES
Supporting School Personnel Following a School-Wide Trauma

A trauma that affects the school campus can be a sudden, unexpected, or unanticipated event that not only disrupts the school's daily functioning but can involve short-term turmoil such as shock, confusion, and fear. Although each student, teacher, parent, or other school community member experiences each crisis differently, a school-wide trauma can have a broad and immediate impact on many children and adults sufficient to interfere with teaching, learning, attendance, and behavior. A trauma that impacts a school can affect a single building or an entire district or community. The following are examples of school-wide traumatic events: an accident on or near the school grounds; a violent incident or crime on campus or near a school that jeopardizes the safety of students and staff; a suicide of a student or staff member; the sudden death of a student, staff member or one of their family members; a natural disaster such as an earthquake, hurricane or tornado; a man-made disaster such as a terrorist attack.

The impact of these traumatic events can be manifested at three distinct levels: the individual (student or staff), the school system, and/or the surrounding school community. The most obvious impact and easiest to identify is physical injury to students or staff. Psychological and cognitive disruptions also occur frequently but may be more difficult to identify. For example, interference with the ability of students and staff to focus on learning is a common reaction to a school-wide traumatic event. Disruptions to the school system frequently occur following a traumatic event, with changes to regular school functions and routines (eg, changes to safety protocols). In addition, traumatic events often raise significant concerns from parents and, when not properly addressed, may prolong disruption of regular school routines. Large-scale events may garner concentrated attention from the community and news media. This attention can lead to prolonged disruptions across the broader community, with repeated exposure to media coverage potentially causing significant trauma-related symptoms in students.

One important role that the mental health professional on campus can play is being part of a multidisciplinary school crisis team, often also composed of a school administrator, school counselors, school psychologists, nurses, lead teachers, a custodian, and other school or district personnel. The team's collective skills can ensure that critical services are provided for the school and the greater community such as assessing the range of crisis interventions needed for a specific crisis situation; limiting the exposure to scenes of trauma, injury, or death; advising and assisting the principal and teachers on how to restore regular school functions and routines as efficiently and quickly as possible; and providing psychological first aid to students.

Psychological First Aid for Schools

Psychological First Aid for Schools (PFA) involves key skills that can be delivered by school staff following a traumatic event to help students acknowledge how the traumatic event has been disruptive to the school environment and to their own emotional equilibrium. By teaching school staff how to respond to students following a trauma, PFA helps stabilize the emotions and behaviors of students, school staff, and parents. PFA also allows students to return to a safe environment and calm routine in an improved psychological and emotional state. Through PFA, students are able to reestablish social connectedness with family, teachers, and peers, as wells as minimize the negative effects of trauma to all involved. The skills students acquire through PFA enable them to identify personal and commonly experienced trauma-related emotions and reactions. PFA can also improve the social support on the school campus, leading to constructive coping behaviors and resilience of students, parents, and teachers, which can ultimately facilitate student attendance and participation in the learning process. Finally, PFA can help establish systems on campus to prepare students and teachers for the future challenges and adjustments that are frequently confronted by schools after a trauma.

The widespread use of PFA is evidenced by the fact that the Inter-Agency Standing Committee (IASC), an international humanitarian assistance forum, has developed Guidelines on Mental Health and Psychosocial Support in Emergency Settings that recommend that "all aid workers provide very basic psychological first aid."[48] The IASC guidelines further define the components of PFA to include, among many others, the following actions:

- Protect survivors from further physical or psychological harm.
- Identify and provide support for those most distressed.
- Reestablish social supports.
- Return to school and familiar routines.
- Facilitate communication among families, students, and community agencies.
- Educate those affected about the expectable psychological responses and basic coping tools for stressful and traumatic events.
- Identify basic practical needs and ensure that these are met.
- Ask for people's concerns and try to address them.
- Encourage participation in normal daily routines (if possible) and use of positive means of coping.
- As appropriate, refer to locally available support mechanisms or to trained clinicians.

Listen, Protect, Connect: An Evidence-Informed Model

In keeping with IASC's guidelines, Listen, Protect, Connect (LPC)[49,50] is a form of PFA strategies focusing on children, parents, families, and community members. LPC uses parents, teachers, primary care providers, and "neighbor-to-neighbor" providers to give basic psychological support. A version of PFA specifically designed for children to be used by educators and other adult staff in schools is available. In the immediate aftermath and during the early phases of recovery, the version, Psychological First Aid for Students and Teachers: Listen, Protect, Connect—Model & Teach, (hereafter, LPC–Model & Teach) is a five-step crisis response strategy designed to reduce the initial distress of students or adults and to help students return to school, stay in school, and resume their learning. The strategy is not a single-session recital of events but a model that can guide the interactions of students and educators over time through the process of recovery. Teachers, counselors, and other adults can use their discretion to apply these guiding principles in a flexible manner.

Step 1: Listen

During step one, teachers or adult school staff should provide students with an opportunity to share their experiences and express feelings of worry, anxiety, fear, or other concerns about their safety. Speaking with students can occur one-on-one if a teacher and student find themselves in a relatively private place to talk. Adults should convey interest, empathy, and availability and let students know they are ready to listen. The teacher can open the discussion by acknowledging what has happened, letting students know that it is acceptable to share their experiences, and establishing that the school is a safe place to share their experiences.

Adults should avoid making judgments and predictions such as, "You'll get over it," or, "Only the strong survive." It is important to validate students' life experiences without probing for more details than they are willing to share. Forcing students to go over their experiences in too much detail, especially immediately after the crisis, can retraumatize them and may cause more emotional and psychological distress to themselves and to others who may hear additional details about the event.

Step 2: Protect

For the second step in the LPC–Model & Teach intervention, adults should try to reestablish students' feelings of both physical and emotional safety. Adults can honestly inform students about events surrounding the crisis such as sharing with them information about what is being done in the community and school to keep everyone safe. This information should be provided in a developmentally and age-appropriate manner. In the classroom or around school, adults should maintain structure, stability, and predictability and make efforts to reestablish routines, expectations, and rules. For example, bell schedules should return to normal as soon as possible. If shortened days are required, keep them to a minimum. Traumatized students may experience more confusion with disruption of their school routines including after-school activities and too many changes to their regular schedule. Concerns about separation from parents or caregivers are frequently paramount in children. Parents can help stabilize children's reactions by resuming mealtime, homework, and bedtime routines as well as community or church activities disrupted by the crisis or emergency. It is also important at this phase to protect students from further physical harm or psychological trauma that can occur through their viewing or hearing repetitive media reports on the incident or through bullying by peers at school.

Step 3: Connect
One of the most common reactions to trauma or fear is emotional and social isolation and the sense of loss of social supports. This isolation or loss can occur automatically without students or adults realizing that they are withdrawing from their teachers or peers. The third objective of LPC–Model & Teach is to help students reestablish their normal social relationships and stay connected to others in order to experience social support. Restoring and building connections promotes stability, recovery, and predictability in students' lives. A student's classroom and school are safe places to begin restoring normalcy during a crisis or disaster. Through the eyes of children, adults can identify the systems of care that are part of their everyday life and move beyond the classroom and school to the family and then to other community "anchors" including preexisting faith and cultural supports. This objective serves to help students reconstitute the relationships between the key community systems or anchors in their lives. Teachers or other school staff who reach out and check in with students on a regular basis can do this reconstitution, sometimes several times a day Students also can be encouraged to interact, share recovery activities, and take on team projects with other students, friends, or teachers. With these types of interactions students feel the caring and consistent support of adults in their lives, even during a difficult time.

Step 4: Model calm and optimistic behavior
Adults can model calm and optimistic behavior in many ways, including the following:

- Maintain level emotions and reactions with students to help them achieve balance.
- Take constructive actions to assure student safety such as engaging in a safety drill to remind them of how to stay safe or planning a project that improves the physical or social climate of the school.
- Express positive thoughts for the future, like, "Recovery from this disaster may take some time, but we'll work on improving the conditions at our school every day."
- Help students cope with day-to-day challenges by thinking aloud with them about ways they can solve their problems.

Step 5: Teach
To support and facilitate the coping process, it is important to help students understand the range of normal stress reactions. School counselors, nurses, psychologists, or social workers can take on this task. They can help students become familiar with the range of normal reactions that can occur immediately after a traumatic event or disaster and teach relevant coping and problem-solving skills.

With early intervention and PFA, the majority of students and adults may be able to resume a new normality of function and routine. However, those with a history of previous exposure to and experience with violence may require follow-up care and treatment for PTSD, depression, severe behavioral disorders, or suicidal ideation.

School staff must be made aware of the risk factors that may indicate a mental health evaluation is warranted. These risks factors include the following:

- Loss of a family member, schoolmate, or friend
- Fear for their lives, observing serious injury or the death of another person
- Family members or friends missing after the event
- Getting sick or becoming hurt due to the event

- Home loss, family move, changes in neighborhood, changes in school, or loss of belongings
- Being unable to evacuate quickly
- Past traumatic experiences or losses
- Pet loss
- Past history of PTSD, anxiety, or mood disorders coupled with any of the previous.

Talking to Parents About PTSD

Parents and other caregivers play an important role in supporting school efforts to help children with PTSD and other sequelae of trauma exposure. In this section the authors highlight information that is most useful to share with parents to help them in supporting the efforts of schools to assist their traumatized children.

When a child is suffering from PTSD or other trauma exposure, it is helpful for parents to understand that their child's behavior can be affected in a variety of ways, not all of which are obviously related to the experience. In preschool-aged children, in addition to the classic symptoms of PTSD, parents may notice the child exhibiting separation anxiety from parents or teachers, regressing in previously mastered stages of development (eg, bedwetting), having difficulty at naptime or bedtime, and having increased physical complaints or new fears. Elementary school–aged children may also exhibit many of these same symptoms, as well as asking questions about death and dying, having more difficulty with authority and overreacting to criticism, being more jumpy, and showing less trust in others. Parents of older children in middle school and high school may also notice their children having more physical complaints and difficulties with authority and criticism, seeming to be more focused on topics of death and dying, and being less optimistic about their own future. Parents of older children should also be aware that their children are at greater risk for using alcohol and illicit drugs.

Parents of children suffering from PTSD or other sequelae of traumatic events can play an important role in supporting school efforts to assist their child by helping to reestablish a sense of safety; providing the opportunity to talk about the experience in a safe, supportive environment; expressing positive thoughts about the future; helping their child cope with day-to-day problems; and providing predictable routines, clear expectations, consistent rules, and immediate feedback.

Parents should also be aware that they can be affected by their child's PTSD, both through helping their child cope with the experience and if the parents were exposed to the same trauma. Sometimes parents find that they cannot stop thinking or dreaming about their child's experience. In other cases parents may have trouble concentrating or sleeping, be more irritable than normal, or find that they are feeling numb or detached. In these situations it is important that the parents seek someone to help with their own feelings.

Clinical Strategies in Working with Students with PTSD

As described previously, evidence-based models for treating childhood PTSD typically include cognitive-behavioral components. The following case example illustrates how you as a clinician could implement these clinical strategies in the context of the school setting.

Case example of Veronica, a middle-school student

Veronica, a 12-year-old middle school student, is referred to you, the school-based mental health clinician, by her language arts teacher. Her teacher explains that

Veronica is typically a conscientious student, especially in language arts, and has a number of friends. Over the last few months, however, Veronica's teacher has noticed that she has begun to miss class, which is negatively impacting her grades. Her teacher reports that she seems withdrawn from her friends, sad, and distracted in class. When the teacher provided minor verbal feedback on an assignment, Veronica became tearful and angry and subsequently asked for a pass to the nurse's office, saying that she felt sick to her stomach.

When you meet with Veronica you ask if she has recently experienced any frightening, difficult, or very stressful events, and she replies that 3 months ago she and her friends witnessed a boy being beaten up and held at gunpoint by a gang in the park. Since then she cannot stop thinking about what happened and worrying that it could happen to her, her friends, or her family and feeling sick to her stomach. She feels upset each time she sees her friends and feels sad and alienated from her peers in general. "How do they expect me to concentrate on grammar and essays when I can't stop thinking about the boy with a bloody face and the gun in the gang member's hand when he spotted us before we ran?"

Engaging and educating parents about trauma

During your initial meeting and assessment with Veronica, you find that she meets criteria for a diagnosis of PTSD. You get permission from her mother to provide her with mental health treatment at school. Although her mother is not aware of this incident, she knows that they live in a neighborhood with gang activity and also shares that the family has been struggling financially since her husband lost his job last year. She also reports that Veronica has been more sad and tired, has been asking for medicine to calm her stomach over the last few months, easily loses her patience with siblings, and does not like to go to school. She agrees that she would like Veronica to receive support and learn coping skills so she can feel better. Her mother works two jobs and has two younger children, making it feel impossible to accompany Veronica or provide transportation for services, so she is grateful that she can receive such services at school and free of charge. While you have her on the phone, you provide Veronica's mother with brief information about the treatment components likely to be included in your work with Veronica and convey that it will be helpful to have her mother involved to the extent possible. She agrees to do her best to get time off to attend 1 to 2 sessions and to support Veronica's practice of coping skills at home as she progresses through treatment. You give her your contact information and ask her to provide you with any alternative contact information for her and best times to contact her if needed.

Creative approaches to communicating with parents can help overcome obstacles to parents coming to the school for sessions. Information may be conveyed via telephone calls, notes or treatment materials passed back and forth, or the child sharing and demonstrating treatment elements for parents and caregivers. If parents transport their children to or from school, caregivers may be able to catch parents at drop-off or pick-up times or arrange in advance to meet briefly during those times. It is also helpful to identify times when parents may already be on campus, such as for a school assembly, evening performance, open house, or school-wide parent meeting. For example, you could arrange to meet with Veronica's mother, on one of her days off just after drop-off.

With Veronica's mother you review common reactions to stress and trauma; have her engage in the same relaxation training exercises you do with Veronica; discuss the link between thoughts, feelings and behaviors and the rationale for the PTSD treatment; and review problem-solving. You highlight the issue of avoidance and why it is important for youth to be able to process and digest their traumatic experiences by telling their stories. You emphasize that Veronica will be practicing skills between sessions at home and may need support in doing so, especially as she works toward getting back to doing things that she may have been avoiding.

Treatment rationale and psychoeducation

One way to convey the rationale for cognitive-behavioral intervention for PTSD to students is to create a triangle with thoughts, feelings, and behaviors at each of the corners and discuss that scary or traumatic events affect everything about us—all three of these things—and provide an example of how they are linked and affect each other. For example, given the experience that Veronica has had, she can see how she now *thinks* that if she goes to the park with her friends or family one of them could get beaten up or shot, and that makes her *feel* very nervous and afraid so she does not hang out with friends any more near the park or want her family to go out of the house (*behavior*). You validate that those thoughts and feelings and behaviors make sense given what Veronica has been through. You can impart the idea that the intervention you are providing helps students who have been through difficult things like Veronica has to think and feel and act in a way that makes them feel better so they can get back to doing what they like and need to do that is safe.

You ask Veronica about the goals she has for treatment and agree together on a treatment plan including information about the different treatment components so that Veronica knows what to expect. You provide Veronica with information about common reactions to stress and trauma and explore what symptoms have been coming up for her and the hope for how treatment may help it improve. For example, Veronica offers that she has not wanted to go places or see people that remind her of what happened. You state that "avoidance is common and makes sense because you may feel better for the moment, but just like not wanting to talk or think about the trauma, avoiding situations or people that remind you of the gang incident in the park can keep you from doing normal things that are an important part of your life, right? In treatment, we'll learn about how to cope with some of these bad feelings so you can get back to doing those things."

You ask Veronica to share a worksheet on common reactions to stress and trauma with her mother and to share some of the symptoms she has been experiencing. You leave a space where her mother can add any comments or questions that Veronica can bring back to you.

Relaxation training

Teaching different forms of relaxation training such as deep breathing, progressive muscle relaxation, positive imagery, and/or mindfulness can help students with affect regulation as they manage their PTSD symptoms. Moreover, relaxation is an easy skill to transfer over to the classroom setting and for young people to practice in the classroom and at home when they are struggling with anxiety, frustration, or irritability/anger.

You explain to Veronica the idea of a feeling thermometer (0–10; where 0 is feeling okay and 10 is feeling very, very upset/anxious/scared) and ask for ratings before and after the relaxation exercises. Veronica is asked to practice the different relaxation techniques during the week and to teach her mom how to do them with her at home, if possible. Veronica quickly recognizes that relaxation could also be something she could try when her stomach is bothering her at school before asking for a pass to go to the bathroom or the nurse's office.

Cognitive restructuring

Cognitive restructuring for children and adolescents with PTSD focuses on ways in which the experience of traumatic events may have affected the young person's cognitions about himself or herself, other people, and the world around him/her. These negative or threat cognitions can generalize to many people and situations, which can lead to a great deal of functional impairment in school, socially, and within the family. It is important to allow students to practice first being aware of the automatic thoughts that they have in various situations (including those that are anxiety-provoking) and how those thoughts can fuel their feelings and actions. Then students can practice replacing negative thoughts with more helpful and accurate thoughts and logging situations where they are able to do so between sessions. You can ask students to write down a couple of helpful thoughts on a small card to carry with them and pull out in situations when their thoughts may be getting in their way.

Veronica became so familiar with these statements that she would just touch the card inside her pocket to remind herself to check her thoughts and see if she needed to replace them with a more helpful or realistic thought.

Trauma narrative

Developing a narrative of children's' traumatic experience enables them to process and digest their story and what they have been through. It is not uncommon that this opportunity in treatment is the first the child has had to recount the story. The trauma narrative can be done in writing and/or pictures and then read and processed aloud, or it can be a verbal recounting of the trauma memory. In either case it is important that the child is able to tell or review the story several times in order to decrease the amount of anxiety that the trauma memory provokes. Explaining that being able to talk about what happened and work through some of the thoughts and feelings associated with parts of the story as it was happening and in the present can make it less difficult to think or talk about what happened. As a clinician, you are able to bear witness to the child's memory of the experience, providing support and assistance in reframing some maladaptive thoughts about what happened and the child's role in it. You will need to determine the number of sessions to focus on the trauma narrative, but you typically do not want it to be more than a third of the total sessions so that many sessions focus on the present and skill-building for the future.

By the second session of the trauma narrative with Veronica, she has created some drawings and narrated her traumatic experience several times, and it is much easier for her to talk about what she went through. Veronica thinks that she is ready to share her story with her mother. You help her think through and plan a good time to talk to her mother and role-play how it might go. You let her know that you will be calling her mom to give her an update on Veronica's progress and that you will talk to her mom about how to be supportive if/when Veronica shares the story with her. You also offer to invite her mother to join you for a session the following week in case she does not find a time to do it herself during the week or after Veronica has shared the information. You encourage Veronica to do something fun during the week to take care of herself, because she has been working through difficult issues.

In vivo gradual exposure to trauma reminders

The in vivo gradual exposure to trauma reminders component focuses on the creation of a hierarchical list of things that the student may be avoiding since their traumatic event. Students make a list of what they have been avoiding that they would like to be able to do again, and you assist them in refining a hierarchy of gradual approach steps, getting feeling-thermometer ratings for each of the steps. Each week you can assist the student in selecting one to two things that can feasibly be practiced over the next week that are rated at 3 to 4 or lower on their feeling thermometer. Typically, once students gain mastery over the items lower on their list, they are ready to move on to items that were once rated higher. This process is something you want to start by the mid-point in treatment so that there are several weeks of in vivo exposure practice and a sense of accomplishment in moving up the hierarchy.

For example, Veronica has stopped letting her siblings play outside when she cares for them, which is frequently due to her mom's work schedule. After assessing for the safety of having siblings play outside ("Do other children in the neighborhood play outside?" "Did they used to be able to play outside safely?" "Is there a place it is safest to be while playing outside?" "Is it safe to do so during the day/evening/weekends?"), you help Veronica list the following steps for allowing the kids to play outside, and she assigns each a rating of how anxious it will make her feel to do so (at present).

Siblings outside in yard while Veronica is inside (weekdays)	8
Siblings outside in yard with Veronica (weekdays)	6
Siblings outside in yard while Veronica is inside (weekends)	5
Siblings outside in yard with Veronica (weekends)	4
Siblings play outside at cousin's house	3
Imagine siblings playing outside with Veronica supervising	2

Veronica decides that this week she will practice letting her siblings play outside at her cousin's house one to two times. She will also imagine them playing outside with her a few times over the week.

Problem-solving

Teaching problem-solving skills can be a key part of intervening with students with PTSD. Clearly, the physiologic arousal, hypervigilance, increased anger and irritability, and cognitive threat bias associated with PTSD can sometimes lead students to react with increased aggression or impulsivity. Also, given the real problems that children and adolescents may face, taking the time to look at options for handling difficult situations and managing social, academic, or familial problems can be powerful tools that can start having an impact right away.

In sessions covering problem-solving you will again link feelings, thoughts, and actions by working through examples and listing potential actions one could take and making links to the underlying thoughts and feelings. You will want to ascertain the problems that the student may be encountering in daily life. Examples of these types of situations may include someone tagging something bad about the student on the bathroom wall, a teacher yelling at the student, and parents fighting with each other. You then engage the student in brainstorming options/solutions, rating each option in terms of how effective it may be in solving the problem with as few negatives as possible (ie, without hurting anyone or getting in trouble) and selecting potential actions to try for the situation.

Summary

Intervening with traumatized youth on school campuses is a much-needed role for the school mental health consultant. As this article illustrates, there are important roles in terms of working with the school staff and addressing the needs of children and families following a traumatic event. Whether a trauma occurs on the school campus, in the surrounding community, or to individual students and families, teachers and administrators may be uncertain how to best support the affected students. A key role that a mental health professional can play is giving school staff the tools with which to support and refer students who may be suffering with PTSD and other trauma-related mental health conditions. School-based clinicians can and should be aligned with the educational mission of schools. By providing early intervention services to students who have PTSD symptoms, clinicians can not only help in improving the social-emotional well-being of students, but also their academic performance in the classroom.

REFERENCES

1. Centers for Disease Control and Prevention. Youth risk behavior surveillance—United States, 2001. Surveillance summaries. MMWR Morb Mortal Wkly Rep 2001;51:1.
2. Centers for Disease Control and Prevention. Youth risk behavior surveillance—United States, 2003. Surveillance summaries. MMWR Morb Mortal Wkly Rep 2004;53:55.
3. Fitzpatrick KM, Boldizar JP. The prevalence and consequences of exposure to violence among African-American youth. J Am Acad Child Adolesc Psychiatry 1993; 32:424.
4. Jaycox LH, Stein BD, Kataoka SH, et al. Violence exposure, posttraumatic stress disorder, and depressive symptoms among recent immigrant schoolchildren. J Am Acad Child Adolesc Psychiatry 2002;41:1104.
5. Martinez P, Richters JE. The NIMH Community Violence Project: II. Children's distress symptoms associated with violence exposure. Psychiatry 1993;56:22.
6. Singer MI, Anglin TM, Song L, et al. Adolescents' exposure to violence and associated symptoms of psychological trauma. JAMA 1995;273:477.
7. Delaney-Black V, Covington C, Ondersma SJ, et al. Violence exposure, trauma, and IQ and/or reading deficits among urban children. Arch Pediatr Adolesc Med 2002; 156:280.
8. Hurt H, Malmud E, Brodsky NL, et al. Exposure to violence: psychologcal and academic correlates in child witnesses. Arch Pediatr Adolesc Med 2001;155:1351–6.
9. Schwartz D, Proctor LJ. Community violence exposure and children's social adjustment in the school peer group: the mediating roles of emotion regulation and social cognition. J Consult Clin Psychol 2000;68:670.
10. US Department of Health and Human Services. New Freedom Commission on Mental Health: achieving the promise: transforming mental health care in America. Final report. In: US Department of Health and Human Services. Rockville (MD). US Department of Health and Human Services; 2003.
11. Saigh PA, Bremner JD. The history of posttraumatic stress disorder. Needham Heights (MA): Allyn & Bacon; 1999.
12. Stein BD, Zima BT, Elliott MN, et al. Violence exposure among school-age children in foster care: relationship to distress symptoms. J Am Acad Child Adolesc Psychiatry 2001;40:588.
13. American Psychiatric Association. DSM-5 Development, G 03 posttraumatic stress disorder in preschool children. Available at http://www.dsm5.org/ProposedRevisions/Pages/proposedrevision.aspx?rid=396. Accessed August 27, 2011.
14. Pynoos RS, Steinberg AM, Layne CM, et al. DSM-V PTSD diagnostic criteria for children and adolescents: a developmental perspective and recommendations. J Trauma Stress 2009;22:391–8.
15. American Psychiatric Association. Diagnostic and statistical manual of mental disorders. 4th edition, text revision. Washington, DC: American Psychiatric Association; 2000.

16. Stein BD, Jaycox LH, Kataoka SH, et al. Prevalence of child and adolescent exposure to community violence. Clin Child Fam Psychol Rev 2003;6:247.
17. Finkelhor D. The victimization of children: a developmental perspective. Am J Orthopsychiatry 1995;65:177.
18. Osofsky JD, Wewers S, Hann DM, et al. Chronic community violence: what is happening to our children? Psychiatry 1993;56:36.
19. Kliewer W, Lepore SJ, Oskin D, et al. The role of social and cognitive processes in children's adjustment to community violence. J Consult Clin Psychol 1998;66:199.
20. Overstreet S, Braun S. Exposure to community violence and post-traumatic stress symptoms: mediating factors. Am J Orthopsychiatry 2000;70:263.
21. Kilpatrick DG, Ruggiero KJ, Acierno R, et al. Violence and risk of PTSD, major depression, substance abuse/dependence, and comorbidity: results from the National Survey of Adolescents. J Consult Clin Psychol 2003;71:692.
22. Bell CC, Jenkins EJ. Traumatic stress and children. J Health Care Poor Underserved 1991;2:175.
23. DuRant RH, Altman D, Wolfson M, et al. Exposure to violence and victimization, depression, substance use, and the use of violence by young adolescents. J Pediatr 2000;137:707.
24. Farrell AD, Bruce SE. Impact of exposure to community violence on violent behavior and emotional distress among urban adolescents. J Clin Child Psychol 1992;26:2.
25. Garbarino J, Dubrow N, Kostelny K, et al. Children in danger: coping with the consequences of community violence. San Francisco (CA): Jossey-Bass; 1992.
26. Jenkins EJ, Bell CC. Violence among inner city high school students and post-traumatic stress disorder. In: Friedman S, editor. Anxiety disorders in African Americans. New York: Springer Publishing Co; 1994.
27. Attar BK, Guerra NG, Tolan PH. Neighborhood disadvantage, stressful life events and adjustments in urban elementary-school children. J Clin Child Adolesc Psychol 1994;23:391.
28. DuRant RH, Pendergrast RA, Cadenhead C. Exposure to violence and victimization and fighting behavior by urban black adolescents. J Adolesc Health 1994;15:311.
29. Fitzpatrick KM. Fighting among America's youth: A risk and protective factors approach. J Health Soc Behav 1997;38:131.
30. Gorman–Smith D, Tolan P. The role of exposure to community violence and developmental problems among inner-city youth. Dev Psychopathol 1998;10:101.
31. Cohen JA, Deblinger E, Mannarino AP, et al. A multisite, randomized controlled trial for children with sexual abuse-related PTSD symptoms. J Am Acad Child Adolesc Psychiatry 2004;43:393.
32. Cohen JA, Mannarino AP, Iyengar S. Community treatment of posttraumatic stress disorder for children exposed to intimate partner violence: a randomized controlled trial. Arch Pediatr Adolesc Med 2011;165:16.
33. Amaya-Jackson L, Reynolds V, Murray MC, et al. Cognitive-behavioral treatment for pediatric posttraumatic stress disorder: protocol and application in school and community settings. Cogn Behav Pract 2003;10:204.
34. March JS, Amaya-Jackson L, Murray MC, et al. Cognitive-behavioral psychotherapy for children and adolescents with posttraumatic stress disorder after a single-incident stressor. J Am Acad Child Adolesc Psychiatry 1998;37:585.
35. Najavits LM, Gallop RJ, Weiss RD. Seeking safety therapy for adolescent girls with PTSD and substance use disorder: a randomized controlled trial. J Behav Health Serv Res 2006;33:453.

36. Kataoka SH, Stein BD, Jaycox LH, et al. A school-based mental health program for traumatized Latino immigrant children. J Am Acad Child Adolesc Psychiatry 2003;42: 311.

37. Schultz D, Barnes-Proby D, Chandra A, et al. Toolkit for adapting cognitive behavioral intervention for trauma in schools (CBITS) or supporting students exposed to trauma (SSET) for implementation with youth in foster care. RAND Health Technical Report. Santa Monica (CA): The RAND Corporation; 2010. Available at: http://www.rand.org/pubs/technical_reports/2010/RAND_TR772.pdf. Accessed August 27, 2011.

38. Stein BD, Jaycox LH, Kataoka SH, et al. A mental health intervention for schoolchildren exposed to violence: a randomized controlled trial. JAMA 2003;290:603.

39. Cohen JA, Bukstein O, Walter H, et al. Practice parameters for the assessment and treatment of children and adolescents with posttraumatic stress disorder. J Am Acad Child Adolesc Psychiatry 2010;49:414.

40. Strawn JR, Keeshin BR, DelBello MP, et al. Psychopharmacologic treatment of posttraumatic stress disorder in children and adolescents: a review. J Clin Psychiatry 2010;71:932.

41. Robb AS, Cueva JE, Sporn J, et al. Sertraline treatment of children and adolescents with posttraumatic stress disorder: a double-blind, placebo-controlled trial. J Child Adolesc Psychopharmacol 2010;20:463.

42. Jaycox LH, Cohen JA, Mannarino AP, et al. Children's mental health care following Hurricane Katrina: a field-trial of trauma focused therapies. J Trauma Stress 2010;23: 223.

43. Kataoka S, Jaycox LH, Wong M, et al. Effects on school outcomes in low-income minority youth: preliminary findings from a community-partnered study of a school trauma intervention. Ethnicity & Disease, in press.

44. Jaycox LH, Langley AK, Stein BD, et al. Support for students exposed to trauma: a pilot study. School Ment Health 2009;1:49.

45. Saltzman WR, Pynoos RS, Layne CM, et al. Trauma-and grief-focused intervention for adolescents exposed to community violence: results of a school-based screening and group treatment protocol. Group Dyn 2001;5:291.

46. Layne CM, Saltzman WR, Poppleton L, et al. Effectiveness of a school-based group psychotherapy program for war-exposed adolescents: a randomized controlled trial. J Am Acad Child Adolesc Psychiatry 2008;47:1048.

47. Wolmer L, Hamiel D, Laor N. Preventing children's posttraumatic stress after disaster with teacher-based intervention: a controlled study. J Am Acad Child Adolesc Psychiatry 2011;50:340.

48. Inter-Agency Standing Committee. Checklist for field use. In: Inter-Agency Standing Committee. IASC guidelines on mental health and psychosocial support in emergency settings. Geneva (Switzerland): Inter-Agency Standing Committee; 2008. p. 5–35.

49. Schreiber M, Gurwitch R, Wong M. Listen, protect, connect—model & teach: psychological first aid (PFA) for students and teachers. In: US Department of Education. Readiness and emergency management for schools. Folsom (CA): Technical Assistance Center; 2008.

50. Schreiber M, Gurwitch R, Wong M. Listen, protect, connect—model & teach: psychological first aid (PFA) for students and teachers. In: US Department of Education. Readiness and emergency management for schools. Folsom (CA): Technical Assistance Center; 2006.

Depression in the Classroom: Considerations and Strategies

Alison L. Calear, PhD

KEYWORDS

- Depression • School • Student • Teacher • Strategies
- Prevention

Depression, or unipolar depression, is characterized in both adolescents and adults by a depressed mood, a loss of pleasure and interest in everyday activities, diminished concentration and energy levels, disrupted sleep and eating patterns, feelings of worthlessness, and suicidal thoughts.[1] For a clinical diagnosis to be made, this cluster of symptoms must be present for at least 2 weeks. Dysthymia is a milder and more chronic form of depression, which must be present for at least 1 year in children and adolescents, and includes appetite, sleep, and energy changes as well as low self-esteem, difficulty making decisions, and hopelessness.[1]

In children and adolescents, depressed mood may be exhibited primarily as irritability rather than sadness. According to Lewinsohn, Rohde, and Seeley,[2] the most frequently reported symptom of depression among adolescents is depressed mood, followed by thinking, sleep, and weight difficulties. There are relatively few differences in the presentation of adolescent and adult major depression, although adolescents tend to report feelings of worthlessness and guilt more than adults.[2]

EPIDEMIOLOGY

Major depression often begins in adolescence, with a marked increase in prevalence between 15 and 18 years.[3] The risk of developing a depressive episode increases with age during adolescence, with the reported rates of depression comparable to the lifetime prevalence rates observed in the adult population.[2,3] The one year prevalence rate of major depression among the child and adolescent population is 1% to 8%, with up to 28% of young people experiencing an episode of major depression by the age of 19 years.[2,4–6] However, these figures may be an underestimation of the true extent of emotional difficulties in the community, with many children and adolescents exhibiting elevated, but subclinical, levels of depressive symptoms.[7]

The author has nothing to disclose.
Centre for Mental Health Research, The Australian National University, Building 63, Eggleston Road, Acton, ACT 0200, Australia
E-mail address: Alison.Calear@anu.edu.au

MORBIDITY

Depression is among the major causes of morbidity among children and adolescents, with the disorder often taking a chronic, recurrent, and episodic course.[8] Some of the negative outcomes associated with depression include family and social dysfunction, physical ill health, poor academic performance, low self-esteem, increased psychopathology, and suicide.[2,8] Depression can be comorbid with a number or other psychiatric conditions, including anxiety, attention deficit hyperactivity disorder, conduct disorder, and substance use disorders.[9,10]

SCHOOL-BASED PREVENTION AND EARLY INTERVENTION FOR DEPRESSION

Most prevention efforts with children and adolescents occur in the school environment. The school system has been identified as an ideal setting for the implementation of prevention and early intervention programs for depression, due to its unparalleled contact with youth.[11] The school environment provides the opportunity to target all individuals—those with depression that has not been identified, those at risk because of stressors or internal vulnerabilities, those with subthreshold symptoms, and those who are asymptomatic but who may develop symptoms in the future.

With the incidence of unidentified and untreated depression so high, the inclusion of these programs in schools could help to alleviate the symptoms of affected students, and provide them with a means to seek further assistance and support. School-based prevention and early intervention programs could also be beneficial to those children and adolescents who are not symptomatic. These programs could further strengthen the resilience and coping skills possessed by these students, as well as make them more aware, and tolerant, of mental health problems in the community.[12]

EVIDENCE-BASED PREVENTION PROGRAMS

Three types of prevention programs—universal, indicated, and selective—have been delivered in schools to prevent depressive symptoms.[13] Universal prevention programs are delivered to all students in a given population regardless of symptom level and are often designed to enhance general mental health or build resiliency. Selective prevention programs target children and adolescents who are at risk of developing depression by virtue of particular risk factors such as parental divorce or depression, whereas indicated programs target young people with early or mild symptoms of depression.[13]

In a recent review by Calear and Christensen,[14] 42 randomized, controlled trials pertaining to 28 individual school-based depression prevention programs were identified. A large proportion of the programs identified in the review were delivered by a mental health professional or graduate student, were 8 to 12 sessions long and were based on cognitive–behavioral therapy. Other common therapeutic techniques included psychoeducation and interpersonal therapy; program leaders included classroom teachers and nurses in some programs. Just over half of the identified trials included adolescents as the target audience and were universal in nature.

Overall, 23 of the 42 (55%) trials identified in the review reported significant reductions in participants' symptoms of depression at postintervention or follow-up. Effect sizes for these trials ranged from 0.21 to 1.40.[14] Indicated prevention programs were found to be the most effective type of school-based intervention, compared with universal and selective school-based programs. Trials utilizing teacher program leaders generally had smaller and fewer significant effects than trials led by mental health professionals or graduate students. The review concluded that there is some support for the implementation of depression prevention programs in schools and that these programs should continue to be implemented in schools as a means of preventing the onset of depression in children and adolescents.[14]

It is apparent from the review that face-to-face depression prevention programs are not always as effective when delivered by classroom teachers.[14] The reason for this finding is not entirely clear, but it could be a reflection of program content, implementation, or training. Nevertheless, it is important to identify ways to improve the delivery of depression prevention programs by classroom teachers, because the delivery of these programs by mental health professionals and graduate students is not sustainable in terms of economic costs or workforce availability. One possible solution to this problem may be the introduction of Internet-based depression prevention programs into the classroom. These programs are currently growing in number and offer a self-directed program that does not require extensive teacher training or expertise to be delivered.[15]

Detailed below is an example of an evidence-based, online depression prevention program, as well as the 3 face-to-face depression prevention programs identified in the review as having the most evidence supporting their effectiveness. **Table 1** presents an overview of these programs.

MoodGYM

The MoodGYM program (available at: www.moodgym.anu.edu.au) is a free, interactive, Internet-based intervention designed to prevent and decrease symptoms of depression in young people. **Table 2** presents an overview of the MoodGYM program. When delivered in the school environment, the MoodGYM program is presented by the classroom teacher during 1 class period a week for 5 weeks. The program is based on cognitive–behavioral therapy, and contains information, animated demonstrations, quizzes, and "homework" exercises. The overall aims of the MoodGYM program are to change dysfunctional thoughts, improve self-esteem and interpersonal relationships, and to teach important life skills, such as relaxation and problem solving.[16] The MoodGYM program has been evaluated as a universal school-based program with young people aged 13 to 17 years. Significant effects of between 0.31 and 0.43 were reported in this study for male depression at postintervention and the 6-month follow-up.[16]

Penn Resiliency Program

The Penn Resiliency Program (PRP) is a 12-session group intervention designed for young people aged 10 to 14 years. The program aims to teach cognitive–behavioral and social problem-solving skills, including cognitive restructuring, assertiveness, and relaxation. The cognitive and problem-solving techniques are taught and applied through group discussions and weekly homework assignments.[17] PRP is among the most widely researched school-based depression prevention programs,[18] with at least 10 school-based randomized controlled trials having been conducted with PRP or a PRP-based program (eg, Aussie Optimism program) since 2001. PRP has been evaluated as a universal, indicated, and selective program, with significant effects reported in at least eight trials at postintervention and/or follow-up, with significant effect sizes ranging from 0.27 to 1.05.[14] PRP has been delivered by classroom teachers, graduate students, and mental health professionals.

Interpersonal Psychotherapy: Adolescent Skills Training

The Interpersonal Psychotherapy: Adolescent Skills Training program is based on interpersonal therapy and aims to prevent depression by teaching social and

Table 1
Overview of 3 evidence-based prevention programs for depression

Program	Age Group (yrs)	Intervention Type	Content	Program Leader	No. of Sessions	Effect Sizes (Cohen's *d*)
PRP	10–14	Universal, indicated, and selective	CBT and problem solving	Classroom teacher, MHP, graduate student	12	0.27–1.05
IPT-AST	11–16	Universal and indicated	IPT and psychoeducation	Graduate student	10	0.31–1.35
SIT	15–18	Universal	CBT	MHP, graduate student, research team	9–13	0.93–1.40

Abbreviations: CBT, cognitive–behavioral therapy; IPT-AST, Interpersonal Psychotherapy-Adolescent Skills Training; MHP, mental health professional; PRP, Penn Resiliency Program; SIT, Stress Inoculation Training.

Table 2
Overview of the MoodGYM program

Module	Description
Feelings	Teaches users how to identify negative thinking patterns, biased perceptions of situations, and negative views about the future. Users are taught the association between thoughts, feelings, and behavior.
Thoughts	Teaches users how to identify dysfunctional thoughts and how to contest and change them. Personal areas of vulnerability are discussed, and there is an introduction to the topic of self-esteem and some basic strategies with which to increase self-esteem.
Unwarping	Teaches users specific ways to change dysfunctional thoughts, with a focus on seeking evidence for warped thoughts and identifying alternatives for them. Further strategies to build self-esteem are discussed, as well as the importance of developing new skills and interests.
Destressing	Teaches users to identify the situations or events that may precipitate negative thinking and the ways in which these situations could be handled better. Stress and stressors and how they can be alleviated are discussed, as well as the impact of parenting styles on negative thoughts. Relaxation techniques are introduced and trialed in this module.
Relationships	Teaches users about relationship breakups and how to cope with them. A simple problem-solving strategy is introduced and demonstrated.

communication skills that are necessary to develop and maintain positive relationships.[19] The program consists of 2 initial individual sessions and 8 weekly, 90-minute group sessions and is targeted at young people aged 11 to 16 years. The group sessions are based on psychoeducation and general skill building surrounding interpersonal role disputes, role transitions, and interpersonal deficits. Program strategies are taught through didactics, games, role plays, and communication analysis.[20] Interpersonal Psychotherapy: Adolescent Skills Training has been evaluated as both a universal and indicated classroom program delivered by graduate students. The results of these trials have been positive, with a significant effect size of 0.31 reported at postintervention for the universal trial[19] and significant effect sizes of between 0.96 and 1.35 reported at postintervention and 3- and 6-month follow-ups in the indicated trial.[20]

Stress Inoculation Training

The Stress Inoculation Training program is based on cognitive–behavioral therapy and provides both individual and group-based sessions for young people aged 15 to 18 years. The program is delivered over 9 to 13 sessions and parallels a 3-phase stress inoculation model: A conceptualization phase, a skill acquisition phase, and a skill application phase. Techniques taught in the Stress Inoculation Training program include cognitive restructuring, problem solving, and relaxation.[21] Stress Inoculation Training has been evaluated in 3 universal school-based trials, 2 of which found significant effects of between 0.93 and 1.40 at postintervention.[21,22] In each of these trials, the program was delivered by either a graduate student, mental health professional, or a member of the research team.

PREVENTION PROGRAM DELIVERY CONSIDERATIONS

The following list of factors should be considered in the establishment of a prevention program in the school environment.

Target Audience

It is important to identify early who the target audience will be—all students (universal), only those students with elevated symptoms of depression (indicated), or only those students identified as being at-risk of developing depression (selective). If an indicated or selective program is to be implemented, then a reliable method of identifying eligible students needs to be determined.[23]

Program Scheduling

It is essential that (a) enough time is scheduled to complete each module or section within a given session and (b) enough sessions are scheduled to allow the program to be completed in its entirety. It is also important to consider when the program will be delivered to students. The program could be delivered in the classroom as part of the school curriculum, or it could be offered as an after-school or lunch-time activity. When a program is delivered is likely to be influenced by the availability of space in the curriculum, the preferences of participating students and their parents (ie, some parents may not want their child withdrawn from core subject areas to participate in the program), and the availability of staff to facilitate the delivery of the program.[23,24]

Support and Protocols for Referral

It is likely that some students will require additional assistance or support during or after the completion of a depression prevention program. It is important therefore to notify the school counseling service of the program's delivery.[23] This will allow the school counseling service to prepare for a possible increase in student referrals or visits. Students should also be made aware of the support services available to them within the school and surrounding area.

Whole School Support

It is essential that the program has the full support of the school executive. The support of the school executive significantly contributes to a program's success in the school environment by ensuring that the required resources (both staffing and material) and support are directed toward the program.[23,24]

TREATING DEPRESSION IN SCHOOLS
Disorder Recognition

Recognizing the signs and symptoms of depression in a student can be difficult, because many of the symptoms are internal and may not be easily identified. Students may withdraw, and this behavior may be missed, or not perceived as being a problem, owing to the nondisruptive nature of this behaviour.[12,25] As a result, it is important that any changes in a student's behavior or general demeanor be noted and closely observed. Students with depression may not ask for help or assistance. This may be because of feelings of embarrassment and shame, a lack of self-awareness or recognition of symptoms, or in younger students, not having the language skills to describe their emotional state.[26] It is important, therefore, that schools assist students with depression by destigmatizing depression and encouraging help-seeking behavior, educating staff, students, and parents on the signs and symptoms of depression, implementing prevention and early intervention programs in the classroom that reduce the incidence of depression, and monitoring students at risk for depression, particularly during stressful times (eg, during examinations).[26]

Box 1
Signs and symptoms of depression in schools
Withdrawn/reduced social behavior
Low mood
Poor school attendance
Impaired concentration and memory skills
Irrational or pessimistic thinking style
Loss of interest
Irritability

IMPACTS ON SCHOOL PERFORMANCE

Children and adolescents exhibiting the symptoms of depression tend to have impaired concentration, memory, recall, problem solving, and physical motor skills, as well as an irrational or pessimistic cognitive style.[7,26] These factors can significantly impact their school performance through reduced motivation, task completion, attendance, work performance, and social interactions. The disordered and negative thinking patterns associated with depression can also influence their perception and interpretation of events, leading to negative views of their environment, self, and future.[27] Children and adolescents experiencing depression may also be less alert or attentive in class, have a heightened sensitivity to criticism, and be more irritable and argumentative[26] (**Box 1**). As a result, it is important that children and adolescents with depression be supported fully in the school environment.

MODIFYING THE SCHOOL ENVIRONMENT FOR DEPRESSION

Depression is treatable and the difficulties associated with this disorder improve with appropriate care and intervention. However, while the young person is recovering a number of modifications can be made to the school environment to assist students experiencing depression. These changes can encourage school attendance and improve academic achievement.

Classroom Modifications

Students with depression may have a seating preference within the classroom. This may be at the front of the class, where they are closer to the teacher for assistance in refocusing or remaining on task, or near the door, so that they can easily leave if they are feeling unwell or are unable to cope. Some students with depression may require frequent breaks to sustain concentration. Seating preferences and breaks, where possible, should be accommodated within the classroom to improve student comfort and learning.

Scheduling Modifications

Depression can be associated with sleep disturbances. As a result, some students may have difficulty waking in the morning or may experience excessive sleepiness at school. This can be accommodated in the school environment by allowing the student to arrive to school late, shortening the student's school day, or scheduling more demanding academic subjects at times when the student is most alert. Scheduling

---

Box 2
Instructional techniques for depression

Develop clear expectations and guidelines.

Provide frequent feedback on progress.

Teach goal setting and monitoring.

Teach problem-solving skills.

Assist the student in developing, organizing and planning their day (eg, use of a diary).

Strategically increase opportunities for positive social interactions with peers (eg, group assignment, small group activity).

Develop a home-school communication system.

Modify classroom tasks, homework or assignments to accommodate mood and energy levels (eg, more time, shorter tasks).

Provide copies of class notes and study sheets before exams to help focus and guide the student's study.

Break large projects into smaller and more manageable tasks and assist the student in planning their time.

Assign tasks one at a time.

Write out instructions on the board.

---

modifications should be revised frequently, with the priority being ongoing school attendance.

Testing Modifications

The test environment may need to be modified to cater for the memory difficulties often associated with depression. This may include multiple-choice formats, rather than open-ended responses, or the provision of more time to complete tests. Scheduling tests for when the student is most alert, or offering alternate testing arrangements (eg, oral examinations), may also be beneficial. All efforts should be made to support the student in their demonstration of what they have learnt.

INSTRUCTIONAL TECHNIQUES FOR DEPRESSION

There are a number of techniques that can be used in the classroom to assist students with depression. These techniques and strategies are presented in **Box 2** and often cater for the student's impairments in concentration, focus, energy, memory, and social functioning.[26]

SUMMARY

Depression is a prevalent and debilitating disorder that can severely affect a young person's social, emotional, and academic functioning. Identifying depression early is essential to reducing the impact of this disorder. Depression is treatable. However, there are a number of classroom and school supports that can be put in place to assist a young person experiencing or recovering from depression. Preventing the development of depression through effective classroom programs should be encouraged and supported within the school environment.

REFERENCES

1. American Psychiatric Association. Diagnostic and statistical manual of mental disorders. 4th edition. Washington (DC): American Psychiatric Association; 2000.
2. Lewinsohn PM, Rohde P, Seeley JR. Major depressive disorder in older adolescents: Prevalence, risk factors, and clinical implications. Clin Psychol Rev 1998;18:765–94.
3. Birmaher B, Ryan ND, Williamson DE, et al. Childhood and adolescent depression: A review of the past 10 years. Part I. J Am Acad Child Adolesc Psychiatry 1996;35: 1427–39.
4. Costello EJ, Mustillo S, Erkanli A, et al. Prevalence and development of psychiatric disorders in childhood and adolescence. Arch Gen Psychiatry 2003;60:837–44.
5. Costello EJ, Pine DS, Hammen C, et al. Development and natural history of mood disorders. Biol Psychiatry 2002;52:529–42.
6. Hankin BL, Abramson LY, Moffitt TE, et al. Development of depression from preadolescence to young adulthood: emerging gender differences in a 10-year longitudinal study. J Abnorm Psychol 1998;107(1):128–40.
7. Bayer JK, Sanson AV. Preventing the development of emotional mental health problems from early childhood: recent advances in the field. International Journal of Mental Health Promotion 2003;5(3):4–16.
8. Merry S, McDowell H, Wild CJ, et al. A randomized placebo-controlled trial of a school-based depression prevention program. J Am Acad Child Adolesc Psychiatry 2004;43:538–47.
9. Angold A, Costello EJ, Erkanli A. Comorbidity. J Child Psychol Psychiatry, 1999;40: 57–87.
10. Fergusson DM, Woodward LJ. Mental health, educational, and social role outcomes of adolescents with depression. Arch Gen Psychiatry 2002;59:225–31.
11. Masia-Warner C, Nangle DW, Hansen DJ. Bringing evidence-based child mental health services to the schools: general issues and specific populations. Education and Treatment of Children 2006;29:165–72.
12. Barrett PM, Pahl KM. School-based intervention: examining a universal approach to anxiety management. Australian Journal of Guidance & Counselling 2006;16:55–75.
13. Mrazek PJ, Haggerty RJ. Reducing risks for mental disorders: frontiers for preventive intervention research. Washington (DC): National Academy Press; 1994.
14. Calear AL, Christensen H. Systematic review of school-based prevention and early intervention programs for depression. J Adolesc 2010;33:429–38.
15. Calear AL, Christensen H. Review of internet-based prevention and treatment programs for anxiety and depression in children and adolescents. Med J Aust, 2010;192: S12–4.
16. Calear AL, Christensen H, Mackinnon A, et al. The YouthMood Project: a cluster randomized controlled trial of an online cognitive-behavioral program with adolescents. J Consult Clin Psychol 2009;77:1021–32.
17. Gillham JE, Reivich KJ, Freres DR, et al. School-based prevention of depressive symptoms: a randomized controlled study of the effectiveness and specificity of the Penn Resiliency Program. J Consult Clin Psychol 2007;75:9–19.
18. Brunwasser SM, Gillham JE, Kim ES. A meta-analytic review of the Penn Resiliency Program's effect on depressive symptoms. J Consult Clin Psychol 2009;77: 1042–54.
19. Horowitz JL, Garber J, Ciesla JA, et al. Prevention of depressive symptoms in adolescents: a randomized trial of cognitive-behavioral and interpersonal prevention programs. J Consult Clin Psychol 2007;75:693–706.

20. Young JF, Mufson L, Davies M. Efficacy of interpersonal psychotherapy: adolescent skills training: an indicated preventive intervention for depression. J Child Psychol Psychiatry 2006;47:1254–62.

21. Hains AA, Ellmann SW. Stress inoculation training as a preventative intervention for high school youths. Journal of Cognitive Psychotherapy: An International Quarterly, 1994;8:219–32.

22. Hains AA. Comparison of cognitive-behavioral stress management techniques with adolescent boys. Journal of Counseling & Development, 1992;70:600–5.

23. Calear AL, Christensen H, Griffiths KM. Internet-based anxiety and depression prevention programs for children and adolescents. In: Bennett-Levy J, Richards DA, Farrand P, et al, editors. Oxford guide to low intensity CBT interventions. Oxford: Oxford University Press; 2010. pp. 393–8.

24. Langley AK, Nadeem E, Kataoka SH, et al. Evidence-based mental health programs in schools: barriers and facilitators of successful implementation. School Mental Health 2010;2:105–13.

25. Tomb M, Hunter L. Prevention of anxiety in children and adolescents in a school setting: the role of school-based practitioners. Children & Schools 2004;26:87–101.

26. Crundwell RM, Kllu K. Understanding and accommodating students with depression in the classroom. Teaching Exceptional Children 2007;40:48–54.

27. Friedberg RD, McClure JM, Wilding L, et al. A cognitive-behavioral skills training group for children experiencing anxious and depressive symptoms: a clinical report with accompanying descriptive data. J Contemp Psychother 2003;33:157–75.

Strategies for Implementing Evidence-Based Psychosocial Interventions for Children with Attention-Deficit/Hyperactivity Disorder

Ricardo B. Eiraldi, PhD[a,b,*], Jennifer A. Mautone, PhD[b],
Thomas J. Power, PhD[a,b]

KEYWORDS

- Attention deficit hyperactivity disorder
- Evidence-based psychosocial interventions
- School intervention

Attention deficit hyperactivity disorder (ADHD) is a highly prevalent, chronic disorder affecting millions of children. Current prevalence estimates range between 5% and 10% of the child and adolescent population in the United States.[1–3] The *Diagnostic and Statistical Manual of Mental Disorders, Fourth Edition, Text Revision (DSM-IV, TR)*[1] defines 3 subtypes of ADHD: ADHD, combined type (ie, elevated symptoms of inattention and hyperactivity/impulsivity); ADHD, predominantly inattentive type (ie, symptoms of inattention in the absence of clinically significant symptoms of hyperactivity/impulsivity), and ADHD, predominantly hyperactive/impulsive type (ie, symptoms of hyperactivity/impulsivity in the absence of symptoms of inattention).

Children with ADHD frequently experience impairment related to academic performance (eg, lower achievement test scores, higher rates of grade retention)[4,5] and social interactions, including strained relationships with parents, siblings, teachers, and peers.[6,7] Because of challenging classroom behavior (eg, significant time off task, frequent rule violations, failure to comply with teacher instructions),[8] teachers often

This project was supported by grant R01MH068290 funded by the National Institute of Mental Health and the Department of Education, K23064080 and R34MH080782 funded by the National Institute of Mental Health, and R40MC08964 funded by the Maternal and Child Health Bureau. The authors have nothing to disclose.

[a] Department of Pediatrics, University of Pennsylvania, Perelman School of Medicine, Philadelphia, PA, USA
[b] Department of Child and Adolescent Psychiatry and Behavioral Sciences, The Children's Hospital of Philadelphia, 3440 Market Street, Philadelphia, PA 19104, USA
* Corresponding author.
E-mail address: eiraldi@mail.med.upenn.edu

spend a significant amount of time providing support to children with ADHD, which may result in conflict in the student-teacher relationship.[6] Also, because of behavioral difficulty at home, children with ADHD frequently have stressful and conflicting interactions with their parents, which negatively impact parent-child relationships and parents' ability to support their children's education.[2] In addition, conflict between families and schools is common among children with ADHD, which further contributes to school problems. This conflict may result from parental dissatisfaction with the teacher's attempts to meet the educational needs of the child as well as teacher concerns about the child's disruptive behavior in the classroom and strained communications with parents.[6] Additionally, parents of children with ADHD often feel less effective in their efforts to support their children's education and feel less welcome in schools compared with the parents of children without ADHD.[9] Thus, because students with ADHD experience considerable educational impairment and challenges relating to parents and teachers, there is a need for a comprehensive intervention plan that targets the child's behavior at home and school, academic performance, and parent-child and family-school relationships.

Treatments to support children with ADHD include pharmacotherapy, most commonly stimulant medication, and psychosocial interventions that are implemented at home and school, including strategies to support family-school collaboration. Psychosocial interventions include strategies to address performance deficits (ie, situations in which the child knows how to perform a particular skill but does not do so consistently) and skills deficits (ie, situations in which the child does not yet posses a skill or performs the skill suboptimally). Interventions aimed at performance deficits include environmental adaptations and accommodations to intervene at the point of performance, such as techniques to modify the antecedents and consequences in the environment to change child behavior.[10] Interventions aimed at skills deficits include direct instruction and increasing opportunities for repeated practice of new skills. The purpose of this report is to describe evidence-based psychosocial interventions (EBIs) targeting both performance and skills deficits that can be applied to address the educational needs of children and adolescents with ADHD. (Readers are directed to key references 2, 10, 13, 16, 17, 23, 41, 47, 55, 66, and 69, for more in-depth information. Resources are provided in **Box 1**.)

SCHOOL INTERVENTION STRATEGIES

In many ways, schools are the ideal setting for the implementation of interventions for ADHD. School-based services are easy to access by children and are provided in a normalized setting in which the stigma often associated with receiving behavioral health services in traditional clinic settings is minimized.[11,12] Schools are the setting of choice for the implementation of EBIs aimed at preventing or minimizing academic, peer-social, and behavior problems, which are common areas of impairment in children with ADHD.

Children with ADHD often do poorly in unstructured and unpredictable environments. A basic recommendation for teachers is to make the classroom environment more structured and more predictable for children with ADHD. As a group, children with symptoms of ADHD are more likely to exhibit disruptive and rule-breaking behavior. These children are less likely to require disciplinary intervention and are more likely to work up to their academic potential when school professionals establish clear behavior rules and a system of consequences that are applied consistently in all areas of the school.

Box 1 Key resources
Schoolwide interventions: OSEP Center on Positive Behavioral Interventions and Supports: Effective School-wide Interventions: www.PBIS.org
Special Accommodations: National Resource Center on AD/HD, Children and Adults with ADHD (CHADD): http://www.chadd.org/
Token Economy/Point Systems: Center for Children and Families: http://ccf.buffalo.edu/pdf/school_daily_report_card.pdf
National Initiative for Healthcare Quality (NIHCQ) – ADHD Toolkit: http://www.nichq.org/resources/adhd_toolkit.html
Social Skills: Children and Adults with ADHD (CHADD): http://www.chadd.org/Content/CHADD/EFParents/SocialSkillsforChildren/default.htm
Behavioral Parent Training: Parent-child interaction therapy (Bell & Eyberg 2002); http://pcit.phhp.ufl.edu
The Incredible Years (Webster-Stratton, 2005); www.incredibleyears.com
Family School Partnerships: Conjoint Behavioral Consultation: Promoting Family-School Connections and Interventions[23]

Schoolwide Strategies

A growing number of schools around the country have been experimenting with school-wide approaches to improving school climate. Some of these programs have been found to be effective in reducing the need for school disciplinary actions, decreasing the incidence of behavior problems, and making schools safer. Two of these approaches are response to intervention[13–15] and effective behavioral supports, or schoolwide positive behavior support,[16–21] referred to as *positive behavior support* (PBS) hereafter. Given its emphasis on targeting school climate, PBS is highlighted.

Positive behavior support

PBS is a service delivery system for prevention and intervention for all children. PBS has been defined as "a systems approach to enhancing the capacity of schools to adopt and sustain the use of effective practices for all students."[19] The practices and systems of PBS are organized along a 3-tiered continuum of prevention with a behavioral theoretical orientation and the empirical foundation of applied behavior analysis. Primary prevention strategies focus on preventing new cases of problem behaviors by using schoolwide (universal) strategies such as schoolwide discipline, classroomwide behavior management, and effective instructional practices. Emphasis is placed on teaching all students key behavioral expectations and routines and creating a proactive means of communication for students and school staff. This is the most common application of PBS. Some PBS programs also offer targeted group-based support for at-risk children (secondary prevention) and individualized support for more severe cases (tertiary prevention).

Use of expert consultants

With some training and support, EBIs for ADHD can be implemented by teachers and behavioral health staff.[22] Expert consultants, such as child and adolescent psychiatrists, school and clinical psychologists, and other behavioral health professionals can play an important role in the deployment of EBIs for ADHD in the school setting. They can assist school districts with the development of systems and mechanisms for the use of EBIs and provide training and support to behavioral health staff. The same approach can be used for ensuring that interventions are implemented in a culturally sensitive manner.

An efficient and cost-effective method that has the potential to affect many schools within a district is the "train the trainer" approach. In this approach, the consultant trains and supervises senior clinicians in the district with the responsibility for providing support to individual behavioral health staff. Some school districts around the country already use similar systems, particularly those that have adapted PBS. In the typical deployment of PBS to a new school, a leadership team is created, and its members are trained and supported throughout the process of developing and implementing universal and targeted interventions in the school. A key member of the PBS leadership team is the PBS coach. The PBS coach, usually a professional who has received training in applied behavior analysis, is responsible for supporting school personnel in the actual implementation of interventions by helping troubleshoot barriers and providing technical assistance. With some modifications to address the needs of children with specific disorders such as ADHD, PBS coaches can be trained to provide support to behavioral health staff and teachers in the implementation of universal and individualized behavioral interventions for the classroom and other areas of the school. For example, the PBS coach could be trained in the use of interventions that address performance and skills deficits that can be implemented in a multitier program to improve school climate and to serve the unique needs of children with ADHD. Similarly, the PBS coach can be trained in the formation of school-home partnerships and the use of conjoint behavioral consultation (CBC). CBC is a structured problem-solving process in which parents and teachers work as partners through the 4 stages of behavioral consultation: (1) problem identification, (2) problem analysis, (3) plan implementation, and (4) plan evaluation.[23] CBC has been found to be effective for externalizing behavior problems at home,[24,25] behavioral control at school,[26] and social skills development with peers as rated by parents and teachers.[27] In this manner, the expert school consultant could have a great impact on the way children with ADHD are supported throughout an entire school district. This type of service could be reimbursed using various federal and state funding mechanisms as well as by research or training grants from federal agencies.[28]

Strategies to Support Individual Students

In addition to PBS strategies, which are designed to address the behavioral performance of all students in the school, teachers of students with ADHD are often charged with the task of adapting classroom routines and expectations to minimize the effects of the individual student's deficits on performance. This is often done via an individualized education plan provided in the context of special education or an individualized service plan under Section 504 of the Rehabilitation Act of 1973,[29] and it involves modifications to routine classroom work, tests and quizzes, and homework assignments for the child with ADHD. Common special accommodations for the classroom include using a modified seating arrangement whereby the child sits closer to the teacher and away from sources of potential environmental distractions, such as doors, windows, or other children with attention problems, and using a private attention cue by the teacher to prompt the student to stay on task.[30] Also, students with ADHD can be given extended time for completing tests or allowed to take tests in a quiet room.[31] Checking assignment books for accuracy and reducing homework load or individualizing homework assignments can also be used.

As a group, children with ADHD lag behind their peers without ADHD in performance and on the acquisition of important skills that affect academic productivity, classroom behavior, and peer relations. Compared with children without ADHD, children with ADHD are more likely to have impaired planning ability, poor sense of time and inaccurate time estimation, lack of effort and motivation, poor self-regulation of emotion, greater problems with frustration tolerance (which results in academic performance problems), disruptive classroom behavior, and peer difficulties.[32] These deficits are generally chronic. Many interventions have proven to be effective, but gains are sustained only if interventions remain in place in the settings and during times when the child experiences difficulties.[32,33] Given that most difficulties experienced by children with ADHD occur because of performance deficits, most interventions are geared toward enhancing performance, such as improving impulse control or time on task.[10] For children who lack skills in the first place, interventions are focused on teaching new skills, such as social and organizational skills.[34] Most effective school-based interventions for ADHD are designed to affect the antecedents or consequences of behavior. An example of an antecedent of a behavior would be the way in which a teacher gives a command to a student.[35] Consequences can be defined as responses that follow a behavior that has the effect of either increasing or decreasing the probability that the behavior will occur again.[35]

Positive reinforcement

There are many interventions that involve a modification of antecedents and consequences. Although many of the interventions based on the modification of antecedents and consequences have traditionally been included in parent training programs, they are also used in schools and can be taught to teachers. These strategies are based in social learning theory and are used to teach teachers how to alter the antecedents and contingencies in the environment to shape child behavior. Many empirically supported programs include components such as (1) setting consistent limits and reasonable expectations, (2) giving instructions in a clear and consistent manner, (3) providing positive reinforcement contingent on appropriate behavior, and (4) using effective and strategic consequences for specifically identified inappropriate behavior.[36] Teachers learn how to set limits and give instructions that are specific, clear, and brief; focus on behaviors that are within the child's control; and develop expectations that are developmentally appropriate for the child.[37,38] Also, a primary goal of behavioral intervention programs is to increase teachers' use of positive reinforcement contingent upon appropriate behavior. Specifically, teachers can provide attention and verbal praise as positive reinforcement when students demonstrate expected behavior and systematically ignore inappropriate behavior (ie, differential attention). Teachers learn that attention, especially when delivered immediately after appropriate behavior (ie, at the "point of performance"), can increase the likelihood of a desired behavior and that the goal of ignoring behavior is to decrease the frequency with which it occurs.

Positive attending (ie, making positive statements in response to appropriate child behavior) is highly useful in strengthening the teacher-child relationship. Because children with ADHD frequently receive negative feedback from teachers because of inappropriate behavior, teacher-child relationships are frequently strained. As teachers learn how to utilize positive attending more regularly, interactions between teachers and children become more positive.

Token economy

Token or point systems require teachers to dispense tokens (eg, poker chips, stickers) or points to any student in the class (as a classwide intervention) or to individual students with ADHD (as an individualized intervention) for exhibiting previously determined behavior. This intervention can be used for increasing on-task behavior or appropriate classroom behavior. The reinforcement can be delivered immediately after the student exhibits the behavior or at another specified time (eg, at the end of a class period). It is very important that the teacher target a very specific skill or behavior as opposed to more general or global behaviors (eg, "raising hand before speaking" as opposed to "behaving well in class"). This intervention is more effective when it is paired with a reinforcement system in which the student can exchange tokens or points for preferred activities or small prizes. Also, the token/point system intervention is more effective when the child is given the opportunity to choose from a menu of reinforcements and when the system is consistently implemented by teachers.[10,39] Some children with ADHD respond to the token/point system only when the intervention combines positive reinforcement and response cost.[40] In this variation of the token/point system, the child can earn points or other reinforcers for exhibiting a specified desirable behavior but loses them when he exhibits a specified undesirable behavior. This combination is effective because it offers the child the opportunity to earn back lost tokens/points by exhibiting the desirable behavior.

Daily report card

The daily report card (DRC) is a behavioral intervention with strong research support[41,42] that can be developed using the CBC model. This intervention requires planning that involves the school and the family with input from the child, implementation with elements involving the teacher and parents, and evaluation of implementation quality and outcomes. (See **Box 2** for guidelines related to developing a DRC.) As indicated in step 5, monitoring quality of implementation and child progress toward behavioral goals are important components of the intervention process. When the DRC intervention is not implemented properly, its effectiveness can be compromised.[41,42] Implementation quality can be monitored by reviewing completed DRCs on a periodic basis to determine (1) whether it has been completed by teachers each day, (2) whether the child has delivered the DRC to the parents each day, (3) whether the parents evaluated child performance in relationship to an established goal, and (4) whether reinforcers have been administered as planned. With regard to monitoring outcomes, a strategy that is easy to use is to keep track of the number of points earned by the child on the DRC each day or calculate the percentage of days for which the child attains his or her goal. For cases in which implementation quality of the DRC in the home setting is inconsistent, it may be possible to conduct the evaluation and reinforcement phases of the intervention at school.

Considerable evidence supports the effectiveness of the DRC intervention with children who have ADHD and related behavioral problems. In addition, the DRC has been found to be an intervention approach that is highly acceptable and feasible for teachers.

Self-management

Self-management, which includes self-monitoring and self-reinforcement, can be an effective intervention for maintaining and generalizing behavioral gains made through the use of the token/point system, especially for older children.[43–45] In this intervention, children are taught to recognize and record instances of on-task behavior after an auditory or visual stimulus at time intervals (eg, a beep from a recording device or

---

Box 2
Constructing a daily report card

Step 1: Identify 2 or 3 target behaviors
- These should be adaptive behaviors for the classroom (eg, "complete work in time allotted") rather than nonadaptive responses (eg, "fails to complete work")
- Consider including the child in the process to increase child investment

Step 2: Identify a method for recording child behavior
- Option 1: Tally the occurrence of target behavior (this option is more challenging for teachers— consider feasibility issues)
- Option 2: Rate the child's behavior on a 3- or 4-point scale at designated times (eg, 0 = met goals 0%–25% of the time to 3 = met goals 75%–100% of the time). Ratings should be given at several times throughout the day (eg, at the end of each class period)

Step 3: Educate parents about the use of the DRC
- Set reasonable goals for child behavior each day. Goals should be about 10% higher than baseline performance
- Reinforce the child for goal attainment. The child might earn privileges at home each time he or she reaches a goal at school

Step 4: Educate the child about the DRC goals; parent, teacher,and child roles; and opportunities for rewards contingent on appropriate behavior

Step 5: Monitor implementation and outcomes
- Review completed DRCs to ensure proper daily use by parents and teachers
- Adjust goals according to child progress

---

a hand signal from the teacher).[39] Initially, the teacher keeps a parallel count of the student's on-task behavior to assess the accuracy of the student's own recording. As the student becomes more accurate in recording the presence of the target behavior, the involvement of the teacher is gradually phased out until the student is in complete control of the intervention. Self-management can be used in conjunction with an incentive system through which the student can reward himself for reaching certain target goals.[39] This intervention can be used to increase on-task behavior but also to improve academic accuracy and organizational skills.[46,47]

Social skills training
There has been a considerable amount of research on the effects of social skills training for children with ADHD.[48,49] For the most part, studies have found that social skills training can be effective but only when it is part of intense, multimodal behavioral interventions focusing on multiple areas of impairment and conducted within the child's social milieu.[50] Traditional social skills training conducted in clinical settings, away from the environments in which these children have relationship problems, lack social validity and, for the most part, result in little to no improvement in social functioning.[10] In contrast, a growing body of evidence shows that partici-pation in the intense programming offered in summer treatment programs (STPs) for children with ADHD, such as the one used in the Multimodal Treatment Study for ADHD,[50] results in long-lasting improvement in behavioral functioning, social skills, and peer relations. These interventions are typically conducted for 6 to 8 hours a day, 5 days a week, for a period of many weeks. The STP interventions involve social skills training followed by coached recreational activities and the use of contigency behavior management systems, such as token/point systems and concurrent home rewards given to the child by the parents for meeting goals related to peer

relations. The behavioral effects of STPs on children's externalizing behavior and peer relations are comparable with those obtained through psychostimulant medication treatment.[45]

Organizational skills training

Children with ADHD frequently have difficulty in organizing materials, which can impact performance at school and at home (eg, failure to bring home materials necessary for homework, failure to return completed assignments to school).[51,52] If children with ADHD do not learn effective organizational skills, they are likely to continue to have difficulties into adulthood, which can impact postsecondary education or employment function.[53] Although medication treatment results in improved organizational skills for some children with ADHD, many children with ADHD who are treated with medication continue to display deficits in this area.[54]

Strategy training involves teaching students academic strategies or skills that can be used to improve academic performance.[55] Most of these interventions target students' ability to take accurate notes, organize their school materials, and organize their study time more efficiently.[55,56] Organizational skills training aims at giving the student more responsibility and a sense of ownership of academic performance and lessening the involvement of teachers and parents. These interventions have been developed in recognition of the increased demands placed on middle school and high school students to understand and synthesize materials from classroom lectures in multiple subjects.[57] For example, studies have been conducted with adolescents with ADHD in which they were taught how to take notes during classroom lectures, how to write down homework assignments with accuracy, how to organize their school binders and other school materials, and how to memorize information to help them study for tests and exams.[58] As with other interventions for students with ADHD, the effectiveness of organizational skills training is enhanced through the use of contingency reinforcement.

Behavioral homework interventions

These interventions are designed to address problems with homework completion, which are highly prevalent among children with ADHD.[52,59] Homework is a fruitful target for intervention because improving homework performance has the potential to improve the family-school relationship and contribute to academic success.

Homework interventions have 2 primary elements: antecedent strategies that create the context for homework performance and consequences, which refer to the contingencies of homework behavior. Antecedent strategies include teacher assignment of a reasonable amount of homework given the child's age, developmental ability, and attention skills, as well as teacher assignment of work that can be completed by the child with minimal parental instruction and supervision (ie, reinforcement learning, not new skill acquisition). Antecedent strategies also involve establishing a place for homework that is relatively free from distraction and delineating a time for homework that is responsive to times of the day during which children are most attentive and parents are able to monitor homework carefully.[60]

Homework strategies that address both the antecedents and consequences of homework are goal setting and contingency contracting.[61,62] These strategies have multiple steps. First, when it is time for homework, the parent and child review together the assignments and break up the work into manageable subunits that can be completed before taking a brief break. The length of the subunits might vary from 5 minutes for a first grader to 20 minutes for a fifth grader, although this assumes a relatively good attention span. Second, the parent and child select the first subunit to work on, which is typically an assignment that is relatively easy for the child, which helps to build momentum for completing other assignments. Before working on the subunit, the parent and child look over the assignment and mutually identify reasonable goals for number of problems to be completed, number of correct responses, and amount of time.

Third, before beginning each assignment, the parent checks to make sure the child understands the directions and knows how to complete the task. Then, the parent sets a timer and the child begins work. While the child is working, it is important for the parent to monitor child performance carefully, reinforce attention and effort periodically, and refrain from reinforcing avoidant or inattention behavior. Fourth, when the time has expired, the parent and child evaluate work completion and accuracy and compare performance to goals. If the child reaches the goals, he or she earns points that can be exchanged later for privileges. If the child fails to achieve the goal, or achieves accuracy but does not complete all the work, the child is requested to move to the next assignment and not go back over the work. In this way, all the homework assignments can be completed in a reasonable amount of time. In these cases, it is important for the parent to communicate with the teacher so that the child is rewarded for effort and does not get penalized for incomplete work.

Computer-assisted instruction
Children with ADHD frequently exhibit academic skills deficits, including problems with comprehension and retrieval of basic facts. If tasks are novel and stimulating, structured to match the child's individual instructional level, and children receive regular feedback about their performance[29,63] then children with ADHD tend to exhibit increased academic success. Computer-assisted instruction is one strategy that may provide the necessary conditions for supporting the academic skills development of children with ADHD.[64,65] Computer-assisted instruction allows for lessons and specific goals to be tailored to each child's instructional level, the learning environment tends to be more stimulating than typical paper and pencil classroom tasks, and children receive immediate feedback from the computer about the accuracy of their responses.[64]

SPECIAL CONSIDERATIONS

Most of the intervention strategies described in this article are appropriate for elementary-age children with ADHD, reflecting the preponderance of research conducted with this age group. Less research has been conducted with preschool-age children and even less with adolescents who have ADHD. Several factors are important to consider when developing or adapting interventions for preschool and adolescent youth.

For preschoolers, a useful strategy to strengthen the parent-child relationship or the teacher-student relationship is for parents or teachers to engage children in nondirective play, which involves carefully observing the child's play, refraining from making directive statements, and affirming creative elements of the play.[66] When using reinforcement strategies with this age group, it is especially important to administer reinforcers as soon as possible after the desired behavior occurs and to do so using salient, concrete reinforcers. If response cost is used as a method of punishment (eg, taking away a desired toy), the duration of withdrawal required is typically very brief to be effective.[67]

For adolescents, strengthening the parent-child or teacher-student relationship might involve giving the youth a chance to "show-and-tell" about an exciting event and listening carefully. When designing goal setting strategies and contingency contracts, it is essential to collaborate closely with the youth and negotiate the terms of the arrangement. Points can be administered as reinforcers, and these can be exchanged for privileges administered at a later time (eg, on the weekend). When identifying suitable consequences, it is often helpful to negotiate with the youth up front so they know what to expect when expectations are not met.[68] Organizational interventions have been developed for middle school and high school students with ADHD, and these can be highly effective in completing homework, organizing the school binder, and keeping track of the school schedule.[69] School support in the form of a check-in teacher or guidance counselor can be very helpful in implementing and sustaining organizational interventions.

Schools in the United States have become increasingly diverse during the last 20 years. By the year 2019, it is estimated that ethnic minority students will comprise 50% of the total public school student population.[70] Research has consistently shown that low-income and ethnic minority families are less likely than nonminority families to seek and utilize services for ADHD.[71,72] If these families do initiate treatment, they often are at risk for early termination.[73] Although research assessing the unique effects of culture and socioeconomic status on service utilization is lacking, most investigators agree that assessing families' opinions and attitudes about the causes and the treatment of ADHD is necessary to develop a treatment plan that these families are likely to follow.[74] Also, low-income and ethnic minority families may be more likely to stay in treatment if they are involved in the development and implementation of the interventions. A strategy that is appropriate for use by school behavioral health staff and that involves families is the formation of school-home partnerships.[75] A partnership approach, such as CBC (described above), greatly facilitates the adoption of culturally sensitive interventions, because the parent, who is given equal standing in the relationship with school personnel, can contribute to the development of interventions that are congruent with their expectations about treatment and school goals.[23,75,76] The use of school-home partnerships is not common outside demonstration projects, and few behavioral health staff members have been trained in the use of CBC. However, this and other promising models of service delivery could be deployed more widely in school settings to great positive effect with the aid of expert consultants.

Pharmacologic interventions, including stimulants and some nonstimulant options, such as atomoxetine, are effective in the treatment of ADHD. Although medication alone can be effective in treating the symptoms and impairments associated with ADHD, there often is an advantage to combining medication with behavioral intervention, especially with regard to improving areas of impaired executive functioning.[77] Further, families typically view medication as an acceptable form of intervention when it is used in combination with behavior therapy.[78] The selection of an initial approach to treatment (ie, medication alone, behavior therapy alone, combined treatment) is based on shared decision making involving the family, school professionals, and the health care team, taking into consideration the child's likelihood of responding favorably, potential for adverse effects, treatment history, and family beliefs and preferences for intervention. Subsequent decisions (eg, decision to combine medication with behavior therapy) is based on response to previous attempts at treatment and family beliefs, which can vary during the course of intervention.[79]

SUMMARY

An extensive amount of research has demonstrated the effectiveness of psychosocial interventions for children with ADHD. Historically, the research has focused on interventions targeting problems in the home or school setting, but more recent research has highlighted the importance of family-school partnerships and conjoint approaches to intervention involving family and school. Effective approaches to psychosocial intervention consist of strategies to address performance deficits, promote adaptive behavior, and improve children's self-control and academic and social skills. Although most of the research has focused on interventions for elementary-age children, there is an increasing emphasis on developing and validating approaches for younger and older children. With preschoolers there is greater emphasis on addressing performance deficits, and with adolescents there is increased emphasis on skill building and generalization of skills across settings. In addition, there is a strong need to adapt psychosocial interventions so that they are meaningful and acceptable to families of diverse ethnic backgrounds; fostering strong family-school partnerships is a key strategy for developing culturally effective psychosocial interventions for ADHD. Finally, given the abundance of evidence supporting the effectiveness of medication as well as psychosocial treatments for ADHD, integrating both approaches to interventions is often the optimal approach. There is considerable evidence to indicate that combined approaches are more effective in reducing ADHD symptoms and related academic and social impairments than separate treatments.

REFERENCES

1. American Psychiatric Association. Diagnostic and statistical manual of mental disorders, 4th edition. Washington, DC, 2000.
2. *Barkley RA. Attention deficit hyperactivity disorder: a handbook for diagnosis and treatment, 3rd edition. New York: Guilford Press; 2006.
3. Polanczyk G, Silva de Lima M, Horta BL, et al. The worldwide prevalence of ADHD: a systematic review and metaregression analysis. Am J Psychiatry 2007;164: 942–48.
4. Barkley RA, DuPaul GJ, McMurray MB. Comprehensive evaluation of attention-deficit disorder with and without hyperactivity as defined by research criteria. J Consult Clin Psychol 1990;58:775–89.
5. Marshall RM, Hynd GW, Handwerk MJ, et al. Academic underachievement in ADHD subtypes. J Learn Disabil 1997;30:635–42.
6. Greene RW, Beszterczey SK, Katzenstein T, et al. Are students with ADHD more stressful to teach? Patterns of teacher stress in an elementary school sample. J Emot Behav Disord 2002;10:79–89.
7. Johnston C, Mash EJ: Families of children with attention-deficit/hyperactivity disorder: Review and recommendations for future research. Clin Child Family Psychol Rev 2001;4:183–207.
8. Atkins MS, Pelham WE, Licht MH. The Differential validity of teacher ratings of inattention, overactivity, and aggression. J Abnorm Child Psychol 1989;17: 423–35.
9. Rogers MA, Wiener J, Marton I, et al. Parental involvement in children's learning: comparing parents of children with and without attention-deficit/hyperactivity disorder (ADHD). J School Psychol 2009;47:167–85.
10. *Pelham WE, Fabiano GA. Evidence-based psychosocial treatments for attention-deficit/hyperactivity disorder. J Clin Child Adolesc Psychol 2008;37:184–214.
11. Owens PL, Hoagwood K, Horwitz SM, et al. Barriers to children's mental health services. J Am Acad Child Adolesc Psychiatry 2002;41:731–8.
12. Stephan SH, Weist M, Kataoka S, et al. Transformation of children's mental health services: the role of school mental health. Psychiatric Services 2007;58:1330–8.

13. *DuPaul GJ, Stoner G. Interventions for attention deficit hyperactivity disorder. In: Shinn MR, Walker HM, Stoner G, editors. Interventions for achievement and behavior problems in a three-tiered model including RTI. Bethesda, MD: National Association of School Psychologists; 2010. p. 825–48.

14. Jimerson SR, Burns MK, Van Der Heyden AM. Handbook of response to intervention: the science and practice of assessment and intervention. New York, NY: Springer Science+Business Media, LLC; 2007.

15. Sugai G, Horner RH, Gresham F. Behaviorally effective school environments. In: Shinn MR, Walker HM, Stoner G, editors. Interventions for academic and behavior problems 2: preventative and remedial approaches. Bethesda, MD: National Association of School Psychologists; 2002. p. 315–50.

16. *Bradshaw CP, Mitchell MM, Leaf PJ. Examining the effects of schoolwide positive behavioral interventions and supports on student outcomes. Journal of Positive Behavior Interventions 2010;12:133–48.

17. *Horner RH, Sugai G, Smolkowski K, et al. A randomized, wait-list controlled effectiveness trial assessing school-wide positive behavior support in elementary schools. ournal of Positive Behavior Interventions 2009;11:133–44.

18. Kartub DT, Taylor-Greene S, March RE, et al. Reducing hallway noise: a systems approach. Journal of Positive Behavior Interventions 2000;2:179–82.

19. Lewis TJ, Sugai G. Effective behavior support: a systems approach to proactive schoolwide management. Focus on Exceptional Children 1999;31:1–24.

20. Sugai G, Horner R. The evolution of discipline practices: school-wide positive behavior supports. Child Fam Behav Ther 2002;24:23–50.

21. Sugai G, Horner RH, Todd A, et al. School-wide positive behavior support. In: Bambara L, Kern L, editors. Individualized supports for students with problem behaviors: designing positive behavior plans. New York, NY: Guilford Press; 2005. p. 359–70.

22. Rappaport N, Osher D, Greenberg-Garrison E, et al. Enhancing collaboration within and across disciplines to advance mental health programs in schools. In: West MD, Evans SW, Lever NA, editors. Handbook of school mental health: advancing practice and research. New York: Kluwer Academic/Plenum Publishers; 2003. p. 107.

23. *Sheridan SM, Kratochwill TR. Conjoint behavioral consultation: promoting family-school connections and interventions, 2nd edition. New York, NY: Springer Science + Business Media; 2008.

24. Illsley SD, Sladeczek IE. Conjoint behavioral consultation: outcome measures beyond the client level. J Educ Psychol Consult 2001;12:397.

25. Kratochwill T, Elliot S, Loitz P, et al: Conjoint consultation using self-administered manual and video-tape parent-teacher training: effects on children challenging behaviors. School Psychology Quarterly 2003;18:269.

26. Wilkinson LA. Supporting the inclusion of a student with Asperger's Syndrome: a case study using conjoint behavioural consultation and self management. Educational Psychology in Practice 2005;21:307–26.

27. Colton DL, Sheridan SM. Conjoint behavioral consultation and social skills training: enhancing the play behaviors of boys with attention deficit hyperactivity disorder. Journal of Educational and Psychological Consultation 1998;9:3–28.

28. Evans SW, Glass-Siegel M, Frank A, et al. Overcoming the challenges of funding school mental health programs. In: Weist MD, Evans SW, Lever NA, editors. Handbook of school mental health: advancing practice and research. New York: Kluwer Academic/Plenum Publishers; 2003. p. 73–86.

29. DuPaul GJ, Stoner G. ADHD in the schools: assessment and intervention strategies. 2nd edition. New York: Guilford; 2003.

30. Parker HC: The ADHD handbook for schools: effective strategies for identifying and teaching students with attention-deficit/hyperactivity disorder. North Branch, MN: Specialty Press, Inc; 2005.
31. Lewandowski L, Lovett B, Parolin R, et al. The effects of extended time on mathematics performance of students with and without attention deficit hyperactivity disorder. Journal of Psychoeducational Assessment 2007;17–28.
32. Barkley RA. Attention deficit hyperactivity disorder: a handbook for diagnosis and treatment, 2nd edition. New York: Guilford Press; 1998.
33. Ingersoll B, Goldstein S. Attention deficit disorder and learning disabilities: realities, myths, and controversial treatments. New York: Double Play; 1993.
34. Langberg JM, Epstein JN, Urbanowicz CM, et al. Efficacy of an organization skills intervention to improve the academic functioning of students with attention-deficit/hyperactivity disorder. School Psychology Quarterly 2008;23:407–17.
35. Tresco KE, Lefler EK, Power TJ. Psychosocial Interventions to improve the school performance of students with attention-deficit/hyperactivity disorder. Mind & Brain, the Journal of Psychiatry 2010;1:69–74.
36. Forehand R, Long N. Parenting the strong-willed child. Chicago, IL: Contemporary Books; 2002.
37. Barkley RA, Edwards GH, Robin AL. Defiant teens: a clinician's manual for assessment and family intervention. New York, NY: Guildford Press; 1999.
38. McMahon RJ, Forehand RL. Helping the noncompliant child: family-based treatment for oppositional behavior, 2nd edition. New York, NY: Guilford; 2003.
39. DuPaul GJ, Helwig JR, Slay PM. Classroom interventions for attention and hyperactivity. In: Bray MA, Kehle TJ, editors. The Oxford handbook of school psychology. New York, NY: Oxford University Press; 2011. p. 428–41.
40. Bilici M, Yildirim F, Kandil S, et al. Double-blind, placebo-controlled study of zinc sulfate in the treatment of attention deficit hyperactivity disorder. Prog Neuropsychopharmacol Biol Psychiatry 2004;28:181–90.
41. *Fabiano GA, Vujnovic RK, Pelham WE, et al. Enhancing the effectiveness of special education programming for children with attention deficit hyperactivity disorder using a daily report card. School Psychology Review 2010;39:219–39.
42. Owens JS, Murphy CE, Richerson L, et al. Science to practice in underserved communities: the effectiveness of school mental health programming. J Clin Child Adolesc Psychol 2008;37:434–47.
43. Drabman RS, Spitalnik R, O'Leary KD. Teaching self-control to disruptive children. J Abnorm Psychol 1973;82:10–6.
44. Dunlap LK, Dunlap G: A self-monitoring package for teaching subtraction with regrouping to students with learning disabilities. J Appl Behav Anal 1989;22:309–14.
45. Rhode G, Morgan DP, Young KR. Generalization and maintenance of treatment gains of behaviorally handicapped students from resource rooms to regular classrooms using self-evaluation procedures. J Appl Behav Anal 1983;16:171–88.
46. Gureasko-Moore S, DuPaul GJ, White GP. Self-management of classroom preparadness and homework: effects on schools functioning of adolescents with attention-deficit/hyperactivity disorder. School Psychol Rev 2007;36:647–64.
47. *Gureasko-Moore S, Dupaul GJ, White GP. The effects of self-management in general education classrooms on the organizational skills of adolescents with ADHD. Behav Modif 2006;30:159–83.
48. Frederick BP, Olmi DJ. Children with attention-deficit/hyperactivity disorder: a review of the literature on social skills deficits. Psychology in the Schools 1994;31:288–96.

49. Pfiffner LJ, McBurnett K. Social skills training with parent generalization: treatment effects for children with attention deficit disorder. J Consult Clin Psychol 1997;65: 749–57.

50. Pelham WE, Fabiano GA, Gnagy EM, et al. The role of summer treatment programs in the context of comprehensive treatment for ADHD. In: Hibbs E, Jensen P, editors. Psychoocial treatments for child and adolescent disorders: empirically based strategies for clinical practice. Washington, DC: APA Press; 2005. p. 377–410.

51. Langberg JM, Arnold LE, Flowers AM, et al. Parent-Reported homework problems in the mta study: evidence for sustained improvement with behavioral treatment. J Clin Child Adolescent Psychol 2010;39:220–33.

52. Power TJ, Werba BE, Watkins MW, et al. Patterns of parent-reported homework problems among ADHD-referred and non-referred children. School Psychology Quarterly 2006;21:13–33.

53. Barkley RA, Murphy KR, Fischer M. ADHD in adults: what the science says. New York: The Guildford Press; 2008.

54. Abikoff H, Nissley-Tsiopinis J, Gallagher R, et al. Effects of MPH-OROS on the organizational, time management, and planning behaviors of children with ADHD. J Am Acad Child Adolesc Psychiatry 2009;48:166–75.

55. *Evans S, Pelham E, Grudberg M. The efficacy of note taking to improve behavior and comprehension of students with attention-deficit hyperactivity disorder. Exceptionality 1995;5:1–17.

56. Langberg JM, Epstein JN, Graham AJ. Organizational-skills interventions in the treatment of ADHD. Expert Rev Neurother 2008;8:1549–61.

57. Spires H, Stone D. The directed notetaking activity: a self-questioning approach. Journal of Reading 1989;33:36–9.

58. Raggi VL, Chronis AM. Interventions to address the academic impairment of children and adolescents with ADHD. Clin Child Fam Psychol Rev 2006;9:85–111.

59. Mautone JA, Lefler EK, Power TJ. Promoting Family and school success for children with ADHD: strengthening relationships while building skills. Theory into Practice 2011;50:43–51.

60. Power TJ, Costigan TE, Leff SS, et al. Assessing ADHD across settings: contributions of behavioral assessment to categorical decision making. J Clin Child Psychol 2001;30:399–412.

61. Kahle AL, Kelley ML. Children's homework problems - a comparison of goal-setting and parent training. Behav Ther 1994;25:275–90.

62. Miller DL, Kelley ML. The use of goal-setting and contingency contracting for improving children's homework performance. Journal of Applied Behavior Analysis 1994;27:73–84.

63. Zentall SS. Research on the educational implications of attention deficit hyperactivity disorder. Exceptional Children 1993;60:143–53.

64. Mautone JA, DuPaul GJ, Jitendra AK. The effects of computer-assisted instruction on the mathematics performance and classroom behavior of children with ADHD. J Atten Disord 2005;9:301–12.

65. Ota KR, DuPaul GJ. Task engagement and mathematics performance in children with attention deficit hyperactivity disorder: effects of supplemental computer instruction. School Psychology Quarterly 2002;17:242–57.

66. *Webster-Stratton C: The incredible years: a training series for the prevention and treatment of conduct problems in young children. In: Hibbs E, Jensen P, editors. Psychosocial treatments for child and adolescent disorders: empirically based strategies for clinical practice, 2nd edition. Washington, DC: American Psychological Association, 2005; p. 507–55.

67. DuPaul GJ, Kern L. Young children with ADHD: early identification and intervention. Washington, DC: American Psychological Association; 2011.
68. Robin AL. Training families with adolescents with ADHD. In: Barkley RA, editor. Attention-deficit hyperactivity disorder: a handbook for diagnosis and treatment, 3rd edition. New York, NY: Guilford Press; 2006. p. 499–546.
69. *Langberg JM. Homework, organization, and planning skills (HOPS) interventions. Bethesda: National Association of School Psychologists; 2011.
70. Hussar WJ, Bailey TM. Actual and projected numbers for enrollment in public elementary and secondary schools, by race/ethnicity: fall 1994 through fall 2019. In: Projections of education statistics to 2019, 38th edition. Washington, DC: U.S. Department of Education, National Center for Education Statistics, Institute of Education Sciences; 2011. p. 34.
71. Burns BJ, Costello EJ, Angold A, et al. Children's mental health service use across service sectors. Health Aff (Millwood) 1995;14:147–59.
72. Kataoka SH, Zhang L, Wells KB. Unmet need for mental health care among U.S. children: variation by ethnicity and insurance status. Am J Psychiatry 2002;159: 1548–55.
73. Kazdin AE, Mazurick JL.Dropping out of child-psychotherapy— distinguishing early and late dropouts over the course of treatment. J Consult Clin Psychol 1994;62: 1069–74.
74. Eiraldi RB, Mazzuca LB, Clarke AT, et al. Service utilization among ethnic minority children with ADHD: a model of help-seeking behavior. Administration and Policy in Mental Health and Mental Health Services Research 2006;33:607–22.
75. Vazquez-Nuttall E, Li C, Kaplan JP. Home-school partnerships with culturally-diverse families: challenges and solutions to school personnel. J Appl School Psychol 2006;22:81–102.
76. Sheridan SM, Kratochwill TR, Bergan JR. Conjoint behavioral consultation: a procedural manual. New York, NY: Plenum Press; 1996.
77. Jensen PS, Hinshaw SP, Swanson JM, et al. Findings from the NIMH multimodal treatment study of ADHD (MPA): implications and applications for primary care providers. J Dev Behav Pediatr 2001;22:60–73.
78. Krain AL, Kendall PC, Power TJ. The role of treatment acceptability in the initiation of treatment for ADHD. J Attention Disord 2005;9:425–34.
79. Power TJ, Soffer SL, Cassano MC, et al. Integrating pharmacological and psychosocial interventions for ADHD: an evidence-based, participatory approach. In: Evans S, Hoza B, editors. Treating attention-deficit/hyperactivity disorder. Kingston, NJ: Civic Research Institute, p. 2–15.

School-Based Interventions for Disruptive Behavior

Terry Lee, MD

KEYWORDS

• Disruptive behavior • Intervention • School • Youth

Defined in various ways, youth disruptive behavior in schools represents a significant concern to youth, educators, caregivers and society. Studies of youth with oppositional defiant disorder (ODD), conduct disorder (CD), attention-deficit/hyperactivity disorder, teacher-identified disruptive behaviors on standardized instruments, persistent early childhood aggression, and negative peer-nominated social rankings all indicate an increased risk for continued disruptive behavior, academic problems, academic failure, peer relation problems, peer rejection, disaffection from teachers, mental health disorders, substance use disorders, aggressive behavior and involvement with the justice system.[1,2] Youth disruptive behavior decreases the time and resources available for teaching and negatively impacts the learning environment for other children, and is cited by teachers as one of the main factors contributing to job dissatisfaction and turnover.[3,4]

The prevalence rates of ODD and CD in epidemiologic studies in United States vary by age, gender, socioeconomic status, community, informants, and version of the *Diagnostic and Statistical Manual* (DSM), with ODD ranging from 2.1% to 15.4% in boys and 1.5% to 15.6% in girls, and CD ranging from 3.9% to 16.0% for boys and 1.2% to 9.2% in girls.[5] The numbers of youth whose behaviors disrupt the classroom go beyond those who meet criteria for ODD or CD.

Disruptive behaviors are often comorbid with other conditions. In general, the presence of comorbid disorders complicates the course of disruptive behavior disorders, and may have implications for treatment.[6] In a meta-analysis of general population studies, ODD/CD comorbidity rates were reported as: Anxiety, 4.8% to 55.3%; attention-deficit/hyperactivity disorder, 3.1% to 41%; and depression, 2.2% to 45.9%.[7] In the National Comorbidity Survey Replication epidemiologic study of adults, the lifetime prevalence of ODD was 10.2% (males, 11.2%; females, 9.2%), with 92.4% meeting criteria for another lifetime DSM-IV disorder, including impulse control (68.2%), anxiety (62.3%), substance use (47.2%), and mood (45.8%).[8] Youth disruptive behaviors draw more attention, but given the high rates of comorbid

Public Behavioral Health and Justice Policy Division, Department of Psychiatry and Behavioral Sciences, University of Washington School of Medicine, 2815 Eastlake Avenue East, Suite 200, Seattle, WA 98102, USA
E-mail address: drterry@uw.edu

Child Adolesc Psychiatric Clin N Am 21 (2012) 161–174
doi:10.1016/j.chc.2011.09.002
1056-4993/12/$ – see front matter © 2012 Elsevier Inc. All rights reserved.

anxiety and depression, it is important for clinicians to assess for co-occurring internalizing disorders.

Disruptive, aggressive and antisocial behaviors have multiple determinants, associated with risk and protective factors.[1,9] Risk and protective factors can be organized around various domains (eg, youth factors, parenting behavior, peers) as well as also static (genetics, prenatal exposures) versus dynamic factors. Dynamic risk factors, which are more amenable to school-based interventions, include the following.

- Youth social-cognitive functioning: Low social skills, bias to attribute hostile intent, hypervigilance to hostile cues, positive regard for aggressive behavior, low verbal functioning, low academic achievement, learning disorders, impulsivity, and hyperactivity.
- Parenting factors: Harsh (punitive and/or aggressive) parenting, inconsistent parenting, low parent warmth, low parent monitoring/involvement, and maltreatment.
- Other caregiver factors: Multiple changes in family composition; parent antisocial behavior, substance use, and/or depression.
- School factors: Poor classroom management, disorganized school, unclear expectations/rules for students, harsh/inconsistent discipline, low reinforcement for positive behaviors, low expectations for achievement, and youth/family low engagement with school.
- Peer influences: Peer rejection, association with antisocial peers.

Protective factors include the opposite of some risk factors, such as socialization with prosocial peers, negative attitudes toward antisocial behavior, youth/family bonding to school, and high parent warmth.

Transactional models of youth disruptive behavior consider the interaction among and evolution of risk and protective factors. In addition to specific parenting behaviors being associated with the development of youth disruptive behaviors, youth behavior has also been shown to affect parenting behavior[10]; that is, youth disruptive behavior and parenting behavior have reciprocal and bidirectional influences. Similar bidirectional interactions occur in school settings between disruptive youth and education personnel. Youth with disruptive behavior are more likely to be viewed negatively by teachers, receive less academic and social teaching, more likely to receive harsh discipline, and less likely to receive positive reinforcement and recognition for positive behavior.[11] Similarly, peer rejection is both a risk factor for and an outcome of youth disruptive behavior. The development and interface of risk and protective factors can interact in various ways. Risk factors leading to low academic achievement, peer rejection, negative attribution style, and disengagement from school can interact and cascade into progressive disruptive behavior, associating with antisocial peers, school failure, antisocial/criminal behavior, substance abuse/dependence, and violence.[1,2,12]

Given the role of schools in socializing and guiding youth, consequences of disruptive behavior in school settings and beyond, and the access afforded by the time youth spend in school, a number of effective school-based interventions for disruptive behavior have been developed and evaluated. Because problems in later adolescence and adulthood, such as school failure, violent behavior, delinquency, criminal behavior, substance dependence, and mental health problems, may be more entrenched and more difficult to treat, as well as share some early childhood risk factors, a number of school-based interventions target early elementary- and preschool-aged children, and schools serving at-risk neighborhoods. The success of public health approaches in medicine has led to 3-tiered, school-based models with primary universal prevention, secondary selected, and tertiary indicated interventions targeting early youth disruptive behavior.

THE GOOD BEHAVIOR GAME

The Good Behavior Game (GBG) is a classroom behavior modification program initially designed to reduce disruptive behavior through a game involving competition for rewards and privileges. Students are divided into heterogeneous teams, and each individual's behavior has potential rewards and consequences for the team. At the beginning of the game, the teacher defines undesired behavior—typically specific disruptive and/or aggressive behaviors—then during a set period of time of classroom activity such as reading or math, the undesired behaviors are tallied. Teams not exceeding the maximum number of undesired behaviors are rewarded; all teams can be rewarded each session of the game. Rewards typically begin with tangible objects, such as stickers, and then evolve to extra activity privileges, such as more recess time. Over time, the classroom spends more time playing the GBG, and the teacher eventually initiates the game unannounced. The goal of the strategy is to encourage students to manage their own and their teammates' behaviors, encourage peer support, and reinforce the absence of undesired behavior. In later adaptations of the GBG, desired behaviors are defined, tallied, and rewarded. The GBG has been adapted and shown to be effective for a number of populations and behaviors. The most studied populations are 1st through 6th graders, but preschoolers, adolescents, and adults have responded to the GBG. Study populations include self-contained classrooms and children qualified for special education services. In multiple studies, the GBG has been shown to markedly reduce disruptive behavior (out-of-seat, calling out, name calling, aggression), increase desired behavior (talking in turn, completing work, raising hands, on-task behavior, good manners), and increase the amount of time for academic teaching while the game is played.[13] In the Baltimore School District, compared with controls, 1st graders engaging in the GBG were rated by teachers as less aggressive and less shy, peer nominations of aggressive behavior among boys were reduced, and classroom observers rated GBG students as increased on on-task performance. This cohort and additional youth were in a longer term study of the GBG in the Baltimore Public Schools. The more aggressive males engaging in the GBG in 1st grade, compared with controls, were noted to have reduced levels of aggression in 6th grade and fewer substance use disorders and antisocial personality disorder at ages 19 to 21.[14]

COMPREHENSIVE PROGRAMS

A number of multicomponent, comprehensive programs to address youth misbehavior have been developed and evaluated. Three evidence-based comprehensive programs are described in this section—the Promoting Alternative THinking Strategies/Fast Track project, Seattle Social Development Project/Raising Healthy Children, and the Incredible Years. The programs have different but related evolutionary pathways, and share theoretical foundations based on disruptive behavior research. Multiple components are used to address the multiple domains and developmental pathways associated disruptive and antisocial behavior. Each of the components has some level of evidence as discrete interventions, and in general the program developers incorporated the most effective approaches to address targeted risk or protective factors. Each of the comprehensive programs seeks to head off later antisocial and aggressive behavior by providing early tiered prevention/intervention services beginning in early elementary school and/or preschool.

PROMOTING ALTERNATIVE THINKING STRATEGIES (PATHS)/FAST TRACK PROGRAM

The Promoting Alternative THinking Strategies (PATHS) curriculum is a universal, teacher-delivered program for promoting emotional and social competencies and reducing aggression and behavior programs in elementary school-aged children while simultaneously enhancing the educational process in the classroom. One of the main goals of PATHS is to prevent or reduce behavioral and emotional problems. The PATHS curriculum is composed of developmentally based lessons, materials, and instructions, and is taught 3 times per week for a minimum of 20 to 30 minutes per day. It includes 131 lessons over a 5-year period that can be used flexibly to target specific goals.

The PATHS lessons are organized around 5 units: Self-control, emotional understanding, positive self-esteem, relationships, and interpersonal solving skills. The components include instruction in identifying and labeling feelings, expressing feelings, assessing the intensity of feelings, managing feelings, understanding the difference between feelings and behaviors, delaying gratification, controlling impulses, reducing stress, self-talk, reading and interpreting social cues, perspective taking, using steps for problem solving and decision making, having a positive attitude toward life, self-awareness, nonverbal communication skills, and verbal communication skills. The curriculum includes strategies activities for skill generalization.[15]

For example, the PATHS Self-Control Unit is a modification of the "Turtle Technique." A series of lessons are presented during the 20 to 30 minutes per day of PATHS curriculum teaching, and accompanied by classroom reinforcers. The students are told a metaphorical story about a young turtle with interpersonal and academic problems, and aggressive behavior owing to "not stopping to think." With the help of a "wise old turtle," the young turtle learns to problem solve by developing self-control. With practice and role playing, children learn to control their negative behavior—going inside of their "shells" when they feel angry, upset, or distressed. Children may be assisted with a cue ("doing turtle") to fold their arms and use a 3-step method for calming down; children then discuss the problem and associated feelings with the teacher. Over time, the "doing turtle" response is shaped for use in appropriate contexts only. Teachers encourage the children to "do turtle" as 1 way to stop and think.[16]

The PATHS curriculum evaluation populations have included general education, special education, deaf/hearing impaired, and preschool students. In controlled trials, compared with controls, students participating in the PATHS curriculum are able to produce more words to express feelings, and demonstrate greater improvements in social problem solving and emotional understanding. PATHS group youth are more likely to offer prosocial solutions to interpersonal conflicts, and less likely to offer aggressive solutions. At the 2-year follow-up, PATHS group youth have been rated as having lower rates of conduct problems and higher adaptive functioning.[15,16]

The Fast Track Program is a comprehensive, multiyear, multicomponent program with a primary goal of preventing severe and chronic problems in high-risk children, identified when they first enter school. In the Fast Track Project, the PATHS curriculum was enhanced with selected evidence-based or promising interventions: Parent training, home visits, social skills training, and academic tutoring to address other risk and protective factors.[17] The program spans grades 1 through 10, and provides more intense services during the risk periods of entry to school and transition to middle school. Two-hour parent and child groups were offered, with attention to parent engagement and addressing barriers to participation (eg, flexible group times, child care provided). Parent groups and facilitators met for approximately 90 minutes while their children participated in separate group social skills training. Parents and their children then met for 30 minutes to practice and consolidate the weekly learning objective. In early elementary school, the parent training emphasized development of a positive family–school link and social learning-based parenting skills that promote positive parent–child interactions and decrease child disruptive behavior. In 5th and 6th grades, the parent group meetings focused on the transition to middle school, preventing substance use and sexual development. From 7th to 10th grades, individual interventions were provided based on risk and protective factors. Home visiting was used to reinforce the group training and address individual youth and family needs.

The Fast Track Project was evaluated in 4 sites: Seattle (WA), Durham (NC), Nashville (TN), and rural Pennsylvania. At-risk neighborhoods were selected based on poverty and crime levels, and schools were randomly assigned to the Fast Track or control conditions. Three successive cohorts were recruited from 1991 to 1993, resulting in a total sample of 891 youth (69% male and 51% African American). Attrition has been relatively low, with 80% of youth still participating after 20 years. Compared with controls, Fast Track children exhibited increased compliance and prosocial behavior by teacher and parent report, and lower rates of aggressive and oppositional behavior by teacher report. Parents participating in Fast Track reported decreased use of physical discipline, exhibited increased warmth by independent observer report, and increased involvement in school by teacher report. Fast Track children displayed higher language arts grades, lower rates of special education service utilization, more positive peer interactions based on observer ratings, higher social preference based on peer ratings, and improved social-cognitive and emotional skills based on child interviews. For the youth identified as highest risk in kindergarten, the Fast Track intervention was found to decrease the rates of all externalizing psychiatric disorders, including CD.[18,19]

THE SEATTLE SOCIAL DEVELOPMENT PROJECT/RAISING HEALTHY CHILDREN

Seeking to improve youth outcomes through increasing prosocial bonds and strengthen attachment and commitment to schools, the Social Development Research Group crafted the Seattle Social Development Project, which was further enhanced as the Raising Healthy Children program. The Seattle Social Development Project (SSDP) is a universal, multicomponent intervention for decreasing disruptive behavior of general and high-risk elementary– and middle school–aged youth. The SSDP provides teacher training, youth social and emotional skills training, and parent training. "Full" and "late" SSDP interventions have been evaluated.

In the SSDP full intervention, teacher training consists of 5 days of in-service training during grades 1 through 6 in proactive classroom management, interactive teaching, and cooperative learning. Proactive classroom management involves establishing classroom routines and consistent behavioral expectations at the beginning of the year. Before school starts, teachers are taught how to provide clear expectations and explicit instructions about attendance, classroom procedures, and student behavior; and recognizing and rewarding attempts to comply. Teachers are also taught methods for maintaining classroom order and minimizing disruptions, providing frequent, specific, and contingent encouragement and praise for student effort and progress. Interactive teaching strategies involve assessing and activating foundation knowledge before teaching, teaching to explicit learning objectives, modeling skills to be learned, frequently monitoring student comprehension as material is presented, and reteaching material when necessary. Cooperative learning entails the use of small, heterogeneous groups of students learning together, and providing team recognition for the group's academic performance.[20]

In the full intervention, SSDP trains 1st-grade teachers in the use of a cognitive and social skills training curriculum that teaches children to think through and use alternative solutions to problems with peers, and avoid aggressive or other problem behaviors. In 6th grade, students in the full and late intervention receive training in skills to recognize and resist problem behaviors, including substance use.

The SSDP provides voluntary parent training. In the full SSDP intervention, when children were in 1st through 3rd grades, parents were offered child behavior management skills and skills for supporting academic development and developing the family–school relationship. In the 5th and 6th grades, both full and late SSDP intervention parents were offered skills training to reduce their children's risk for substance use and other problem behaviors. The curriculum seeks to reduce drug abuse and related problem behavior by helping parents create opportunities for youth to be involved with their families in meaningful ways, strengthen family bonds, set clear behavioral expectations, establish a family policy on drug use, teach their children to resist peer pressure, reduce family conflict and negative feelings, and practice consistent parenting.[20]

SSDP evaluation revealed that white male SSDP students, compared with controls, exhibited lower levels of aggression and externalizing behaviors, whereas white females reported lower levels of self-destructive behaviors based on teacher report. SSDP students reported less initiation of alcohol use and delinquent behavior; increases in positive family management practices, communication, and attachment to family; and more attachment and commitment to school. At the end of 6th grade, high-risk SSDP boys were less involved with antisocial peers. At the end of 11th grade, 5 years after the end of the intervention, SSDP students reported decreased involvement in violent delinquency and sexual activity, less alcohol intoxication, and less drinking and driving. At age 18 years, SSDP full intervention youth reported reduced violent delinquent acts, heavy drinking, engaging in sexual intercourse, multiple sex partners, and pregnancy. The full intervention group reported better academic achievement and less school misbehavior. Youth in the late intervention reported less school misbehavior than controls. At age 21 years, 9 years after the end of the intervention, the SSDP full intervention youth reported better school or work functioning, more optimism about educational and vocational prospects, better emotional regulation, fewer symptoms of social phobia, and fewer thoughts about suicide. The full intervention group was also less likely to be highly involved with crime, sell drugs in the previous year, or receive an official court charge in their life,[21] and less likely to engage in risky sexual practices.[22]

The Raising Health Children (RHC) program utilizes the teacher, parent, and child interventions from SSDP and is enhanced with universal and selected interventions in middle and high schools, including more structured peer activities. In addition, RHC organized schools rather than classrooms as the unit of intervention, to promote a more consistent and global program implementation. RHC emphasizes association with prosocial peers and adults; youth academic, cognitive, and social skills training; reinforcement for engaging in prosocial behaviors; and healthy beliefs and standards regarding substance use.

Children in RHC schools, compared with controls, had higher academic performance and stronger commitment to school based on teacher and parent report, and reduced antisocial behavior and increased social competency based on teacher report.[20] Between 6th and 10th grades, the RHC group had significantly less growth in the frequency of alcohol and marijuana use.[23]

THE INCREDIBLE YEARS

The Incredible Years (IY) is a set of 3 comprehensive, multicomponent, developmentally based curricula for parents, teachers, and children designed to promote emotional and social competencies in young children. The IY Training for Children, or "Dinosaur School," was originally developed to treat clinic-referred children 3 to 7 years old with disruptive behavior. In 2 randomized trials with clinic-referred youth and families, the IY Dinosaur School was found to decrease disruptive behavior both at school and home, by teacher, parent, and independent observation report.[24]

The classroom-based version of the IY Dinosaur Curriculum is designed for children 3 to 8 years old. It consists of 15- to 20-minute large group lesson plans 2 to 3 times per week, followed by small group practice activities. There are more than 300 small group activities and 100 videos to facilitate the teaching of social and problem-solving skills. Students are introduced to Dinosaur School and learn the importance of group rules, such as following directions, keeping hands to oneself, listening to the teacher, and using a polite and friendly voice. Children learn to regulate their emotions and to identify their own as well as others' feelings. Using laminated cue cards and videos of children demonstrating various emotions, students discuss and learn about a wide range of feelings, starting with more basic feelings and then moving to the more complex ones. Children learn to check their bodies and faces for tense or relaxed muscles, frowns or smiles, and other body parts, such as butterflies in their stomachs. Next, children are trained to use their "detective" skills to look for clues in another person's facial expression, behavior, or tone of voice to determine what the other person may be feeling, and why he or she might be feeling that way. As students become more skilled at recognizing feelings in themselves and others, they begin to develop perspective taking, empathy, and emotion regulation. Children also begin to learn strategies for changing negative feelings into more positive feelings. Wally, a child-sized puppet, shares some of his "secrets" for calming down, such as deep breaths or thinking happy thoughts. Role plays are used, including students playing the part of the teacher, parent, or another child to promote perspective taking.

Teachers help students to generate more prosocial solutions, and to evaluate which solutions are likely to lead to positive consequences. Children learn a 7-step process of problem solving: (1) How am I feeling, and what is my problem? (2) What is a solution? (3) What are some more solutions? (4) What are the consequences of the different possible solutions? (5) What is the best solution? (6) Can I use my plan? and (7) How did I do? Laminated cue cards of over 40 pictured solutions are provided in Wally's detective kit as adjunctive tools for solution generation. Students role play solutions to problems introduced by puppets, videos or students themselves. Students are cued to use prosocial solutions from their solution kit when real-life problems emerge. A puppet, Tiny Turtle, teaches a 5-step anger management strategy: (1) Recognize anger, (2) think "stop," (3) take a deep breath, (4) go into your shell and tell yourself "I need to calm down," and (5) try again. Tiny's shell is the basis for multiple activities: Making a large cardboard shell that students can hide under, making grocery bag "shell" vests, making small shells for toy figures who the children help to calm down, and making "teasing shields"—cardboard shields paired with words on cards; friendly words are on cards with Velcro and stick to the shield, whereas unfriendly words have no Velcro and slip off the shield. Children are taught to recognize body clues that they are becoming angry, and to use self-talk, deep breathing, and positive imagery to calm down. Teachers use guided imagery exercises to help students pretend to be in a turtle shell and experience feeling relaxed and calm. Videos of children managing anger or being teased or rejected are used in role plays to practice self-calming techniques. During the role plays, teachers and puppets also help students to change some of their negative attributions. Alternative explanations are offered, such as, "Maybe he bumped you accidentally and not on purpose" or "Maybe he teased you because he really wanted to be your friend but didn't know how to ask you nicely." Molly Manners teaches how to be friendly and how to talk with friends. Students are taught a repertoire of friendly behaviors, such as sharing, trading, taking turns, making a suggestion, apologizing, agreeing with others, and giving compliments. As with other units, the teaching strategies involve modeling friendship skills with puppets and videos, guided practice in role plays and games, coaching skills during small group activities, and promoting skills during the day.[25]

IY Dinosaur School teachers are trained on strategies for developing positive relationships with students and families, proactive teaching methods, effective use of positive reinforcement, incentive programs for targeted prosocial skills, setting up discipline hierarchies, and individual behavior plans for children with identified behavior problems. Parent engagement strategies include invitations for parents to participate in school–home behavior plans, regular letters to parents about Dinosaur School, weekly Dinosaur homework for children to complete with parents, and invitations to visit the classroom.

The IY Dinosaur School curriculum was evaluated in Seattle area Head Start preschools and elementary schools serving low-income and ethnically diverse neighborhoods. Results indicated that Dinosaur School teachers used more positive classroom management strategies and more specific teaching strategies that addressed social and emotional skills compared with control teachers. Classroom observers rated Dinosaur School students as demonstrating more improvement in social competence and emotional self-regulation, and exhibiting fewer disruptive behaviors than controls. Children from classrooms with the greatest initial risk benefitted the most from the intervention. Dinosaur School teachers reported they were more involved and bonded with parents.[24]

In another portion of the same study, combined parent training and the Dinosaur School classroom intervention was compared with the Dinosaur School classroom intervention only. The IY group parent training consists of teaching positive discipline strategies and effective parenting skills, and strategies for improving children's social skills and academic performance. Parents set goals for themselves and group leaders facilitate learning using group discussion, video vignettes, role playing, and home assignments. Parent engagement strategies included providing meals, transportation, childcare, weekly phone reminders, pairing with another parent "buddy," and a small gift certificate for attending a majority of the group sessions.

Mothers in the combined IY parent and Dinosaur intervention were observed by independent raters to have decreased harsh/critical parenting, self-reported more use of praise and incentives, and reported reductions of child externalizing behaviors, and were rated by teachers as being more involved their children's education. There were no differences in teacher reports of child behavior at school between the combined IY parent and classroom intervention and IY classroom only groups, which the authors ascribe to the effectiveness and specificity of the IY classroom intervention—both IY intervention groups had less teacher-reported externalizing problem compared with controls.[26]

ACTIVE INGREDIENTS OF EFFECTIVE SCHOOL-BASED INTERVENTIONS FOR DISRUPTIVE BEHAVIOR

In considering the empirically supported school based interventions for disruptive behavior, a number of significant findings guide contemporary clinical decision making.

- Universal prevention strategies are more likely to reduce the number of children who will develop problem behaviors in the school setting, and are favored over strategies targeted to individual students.
- Child social-cognitive skills training, teacher training, and reinforcing group outcomes provide marked positive effects in the classroom.
- Emotional regulation, anger control, perspective taking/empathy, and problem-solving and social skills training integrated into the general classroom curriculum each show benefit in decreasing disruptive behaviors.
- Teacher training to implement consistent classroom routines and behavioral expectations at the beginning of the school year help ensure that students understand and respond to expectations.
- Positive reinforcements for desired and prosocial behaviors and avoidance of harsh discipline for negative behavior is more effective for children with disruptive behavior. Negative attention and efforts to "break" disruptive behaviors only diminishes student investment in prosocial classroom behaviors, and at best teaches these students to better conceal disruptive behaviors.
- Multiple trials, modalities, trainers, and settings are needed for students to best learn, practice, and extrapolate new skills across environments. Concrete and metaphorical approaches (eg, "turtle-ing" to go inside and think) facilitate learning.
- Heterogeneous peer and small group activities and reinforcement for desired group outcomes improves social and academic skills, promotes positive peer relationships, and increases support networks for at-risk youth.
- Caregiver participation improves family–school communication and facilitates coordination of academic and behavioral efforts. This seems to be critical for high-risk students' long-term outcomes.

BEHAVIORAL ANALYSIS

Given the complexity of youth disruptive behavior, understanding of the purposes or functions of problematic behavior helps to inform intervention development. This approach assumes that behavior can generally be understood (although not always at the time of the event) contrasted with believing that behavior occurs out of the blue or is generally unpredictable. In trying to understand the function of behavior, it can be helpful to consider categories of function. There are various classification systems used, but common behavior function categories include the following: Get attention, get help, get something tangible, get feedback or approval, get power or control, communicate something, outcome of not understanding, escape or avoid a situation, reduce anxiety, reduce boredom, and prevent the interruption of a favored activity. By assessing the sequence of vulnerabilities, setting events, cues/stimuli, problem behavior and outcomes, and the associated thoughts, feelings, and behaviors, possible explanations for problem behavior can be generated.[27] Hypothesis testing may include the development of a specific intervention to alter one of the chain of events, such as removing a cue/stimulus or changing the outcome/consequence. Similar appearing behaviors may have very different functions, which in turn call for different interventions. To illustrate this, some examples of disruptive behaviors, possible functions and potential interventions are listed in **Table 1**.

Table 1
Disruptive behaviors, possible functions, and potential interventions

Behavior	Apparent Function	Intervention
Aggression—child pushes peers on the playground at recess	Get in the front of the line for the slide; youth has difficulty waiting for turn	Teach turn taking and delaying gratification. Practice skills with adults then peers, including target behavior of waiting in line while other children go down the slide. Reinforce practice and using skills in more natural settings. Adults and peers will help cue youth to use skills. Consider assessment for attention-deficit/hyperactivity disorder.
Aggression—child pushes peers on the playground at recess	Child is frustrated with not getting passed the ball at recess, and has difficulty using words to express anger	Anger management to identify when becoming frustrated, learn self-calming techniques to manage angry feelings, and use words to express self and communicate needs. Provide play skills training and also teach getting adult help when frustrated. Involve peer(s) to practice skills, provide reinforcement for youth skillful behavior (tell youth they like being around youth when youth waits turn and is not angry) and increase support for youth. Reinforce peer efforts of inclusion.
Aggression—child pushes peers on the playground at recess	Youth wants to continue playing, and does not want to come in from recess; behavior serves to delay coming in from recess	In simple terms, explain function of various school day activities to youth, and need to stick to schedule. Refer to rules and expectations presented at the beginning of school year. Playground aid will facilitate transition by supportively telling youth when there are 5 and then 1 minute left in recess, and encourage preparing to come in; then support youth in coming in when recess is over. Practice transition with playground aid. Involve peers to encourage and reinforce youth positive transition. Schedule predictable classroom activity after recess that youth, and hopefully most of the other students, enjoy. Develop reinforcement system for appropriately coming in from recess and transitioning to next activity.

Calls out in class	Escape situation, to avoid being called on because of anxiety about speaking in front of class	For anxiety regarding speaking in front of class, assess associated cognitions and teach self-calming technique. Practice being called on and answering with teacher alone, then small groups, and then in class. Teacher may stand closer to student while responding to increase support and so student may concentrate on teacher versus whole class. Develop alternative "escape" behavior for communicating with teacher that student does not wish to be called on—such as raising hand in a certain way. Practice self-calming with teacher, who may later cue youth. Develop token system to reinforce practice and behavior approximating target behavior, and for using alternative "escape" behavior.
Calls out in class	Escape behavior, to avoid assignment youth does not understand	Determine whether academic material is appropriate for youth, and assess whether youth qualifies for additional support. Teach child appropriate ways to communicate not understanding material and how to ask for help. Explain to child that communicating a lack of understanding will be reinforced, not negatively consequenced. Review cues to feeling overwhelmed by material. Practice asking for help and communicating feeling overwhelmed. Teacher to check in frequently to assess level of understanding, and whether more teaching and support indicated.
Out-of-seat behavior	Help seeking	Train child on appropriate ways to get teacher attention and ask for help, such as stay in chair and raise hand. Practice with teacher and other adults, initially responding quickly, then helping child to tolerate waiting longer. Write goal and steps on paper taped on desk for youth to refer to. Develop token system to reinforce skillful behavior.

(continued on next page)

Table 1
(continued)

Behavior	Apparent Function	Intervention
Out-of-seat behavior	Youth seems to be hyperactive and distractible	Discuss possible evaluation for attention-deficit/hyperactivity disorder with family. Break desk tasks into smaller chunks with frequent teacher proximity to assess whether youth is on task; cure and redirect if indicated. Consider use of carrel and/or earphones to decrease stimulation when doing desk work.
Youth not turning in homework	Behavior is a function of youth disorganization and poor school–family link	In a welcoming tone, invite caregivers to come in and discuss youth progress, emphasizing youth outcomes and praising youth and caregiver efforts and skills. Suggest daily report card to facilitate communication, clarify academic expectations, coordinate targeted behaviors and reinforcers, and promote skill generalization.

SUMMARY

Youth disruptive behavior is a concern for youth, school personnel, families, and society. Disruptive behaviors in early childhood negatively impact the classroom environment, and are associated with negative academic, social, behavioral, emotional, substance use, health, and justice system outcomes in adolescence and adulthood. Effective, comprehensive, multicomponent interventions targeting risk/ protective factors and pathways associated with antisocial behavior have been shown to reduce and/or mitigate these negative outcomes. Positive effects have been demonstrated for universal and indicated programs for all participating youth and families in early childhood, and for high-risk youth in adolescence and young adulthood. These empirically supported programs inform the treatment of complex and difficult-to-treat disruptive behavior.

REFERENCES

1. Dodge KA, Pettit GS. A biopsychosoical model of development chronic conduct problems in adolescence. Dev Psychol 2003;39:349–71.
2. Dodge KA, Greenberg MT, Malone PS; The Conduct Problems Prevention Research Group. Testing an idealized dynamic cascade model of the development of serious violence in adolescence. Child Dev 2008;79:1907–27.
3. Ingersoll RM. Teacher turnover and teacher shortages: an organizational analysis. Am Ed Res J 2001;38:499–534.
4. Dinkes R, Cataldi E, Lin-Kelly W, et al. Indicators of school crime and safety: 2007. Washington (DC): National Center for Educational Statistics; 2007.
5. Loeber R, Burke JD, Lahey BB, et al. Oppositional defiant and conduct disorder: a review of the past 10 years, part I. J Am Acad Child Adolesc Psychiatry 2000;39: 1468–84.
6. Hinshaw SP. Academic underachievement, attention deficits, and aggression: comorbidity and implications for treatment. J Consult Clin Psychol 1992;60:893–903.
7. Angold A, Costello EJ, Erkanli A. Comorbidity. J Child Psychol Psychiatry 1999;40: 57–87.
8. Nock MK, Kazdin AE, Hiripi E, et al. Lifetime prevalence, correlates and persistence of oppositional defiant disorder: results from the National Comorbidity Survey Replication. J Child Psychol Psychiatry 2007;48:703–13.
9. Powell NR, Lochman JE, Boxmeyer CL. The prevention of conduct problems. Intl Rev Psychiatry 2007;19:597–605.
10. Burke JD, Pardini DA, Loeber R. Reciprocal relationships between parenting behavior and disruptive psychopathology from childhood through adolescence. J Abnormal Child Psychol 2008;36:679–92.
11. Arnold DH. Co-occurrence of externalizing behavior problems and emergent academic difficulties in young high-risk boys: a preliminary evaluation of patterns and mechanisms. J Appl De Psychology 1997;18:317–30.
12. Conduct Problems Prevention Research Group. The effects of the Fast Track preventive intervention on the development of conduct disorder across childhood. Child Dev 2011;82:331–45.
13. Tingstrom DH, Sterling-Turner HE, Wilczynski SM. The Good Behavior Game: 1969–2002. Behav Mod 2006;30:225–53.
14. Kellam SG, Brown CH, Poduska JM, et al. Effects of a universal classroom behavior management program in first and second grades on young adult behavioral, psychiatric and social outcomes. Drug Alcohol Depend 2008;95(Suppl 1):S5–S28.

15. Greenberg MT, Kusche C, Mihalic SF. Blueprints for Violence Prevention, Book Ten: Promoting alternative thinking strategies (PATHS). Boulder (CO): Center for the Study and Prevention of Violence; 1998.

16. Kam CM, Greenberg MT, Kusche CA. Sustained effects of the PATHS curriculum on the social and psychological adjustment of children in special education. J Emot Behav Disord 2004;12:66–78.

17. Conduct Problems Prevention Research Group. Initial impact of the Fast Track prevention trial for conduct problems: I. the high-risk sample. J Consult Clin Psychol 1999;67:631–47.

18. Conduct Problems Prevention Research Group. Initial impact of the Fast Track prevention trial for conduct problems: II. classroom effects. J Consult Clin Psychol 1999;67:648–57.

19. Conduct Problems Research Group. The effects of the Fast Track preventive intervention on the development of conduct disorder across childhood. Child Dev 2011; 82:331–45.

20. Catalano RF, Haggerty KP, Oesterle S, et al. The importance of bonding to school for healthy development: findings from the Social Development Research Group. J School Health 2004;74:252–61.

21. Hawkins JF, Kosterman R, Catalano RF, et al. Promoting positive adult functioning through social development intervention in childhood. Arch Pediatr Adolesc Med 2004;159:25–31.

22. Lonczak HS, Abbott RD, Hawkins JD, et al. Effects of the Seattle Social Development Project on sexual behavior, pregnancy, birth, and sexually transmitted disease outcomes by age 21 years. Arch Pediatr Adolesc Med 2004;156:438–47.

23. Brown EC, Catalano RF, Fleming KP, et al. Adolescent substance use outcomes in the Raising Healthy Children project: a two-part latent growth curve analysis. J Consult Clin Psychol 2005;73:699–710.

24. Webster-Stratton C, Reid MJ, Stoolmiller M. Preventing conduct problems and improving school readiness: evaluation of the Incredible Years Teacher and Child Training Programs in high-risk schools. J Child Psychol Psychiatry 2008;49:471–88.

25. Webster-Stratton C, Reid MJ. Strengthening social and emotional competence in young children—the foundation for early school readiness and success: Incredible Years classroom social skills and problem-solving curriculum. J Infant Young Children 2004;17:96–113.

26. Reid MJ, Webster-Stratton C, Hammond M. Enhancing a classroom social competence and problem-solving training to families of moderate to high-risk elementary school children. J Clin Child Adolesc Psychol 2007;36:605–20.

27. Miller AL, Rathus JH, Linehan MM. Dialectical behavior therapy with suicidal adolescents. New York: Guilford Press; 2007.

Adolescent Substance Use Disorders in the School Setting

Amy M. Yule, MD[a],*, Jefferson B. Prince, MD[b,c,d]

KEYWORDS

- Substance abuse • Adolescents • Prevention programs
- School • Treatment

Adolescent substance use is a major public health problem that concerns parents, schools, clinicians, and policy makers. Substance use disorders have a lifetime prevalence of 11.4% in 13- to 18-year-olds, with equal numbers of males and females affected.[1] Three national studies: Monitoring the Future, National Survey on Drug Use and Health, and the Youth Risk Behavior Surveillance Survey have tracked adolescent substance use trends. The 2010 Monitoring the Future survey showed that alcohol, marijuana, and cigarettes continue to be the most widely used substances among adolescents.[2] Although the use of alcohol has been declining since peaking in the 1990s, it remains the most common substance used by adolescents, and the prevalence of binge drinking over the past year was 23% in 2010.[2] Marijuana use has been increasing over the past 3 years and reached an annual prevalence of 24.5% of high school students in 2010, with 1 in 16 students using marijuana daily.[2] With the exceptions of marijuana and prescription opiates, the use of illicit drugs by adolescents has been trending down after peaking in the 1990s.[2]

Substance use in adolescence progressively increases with age, and abuse progresses in stages from experimentation to problem use, and later abuse and dependence.[3] Although it is difficult to predict who will progress to problem use, abuse, or dependence, there are identifiable risk factors that indicate level of vulnerability. These risk factors include use before age 14, family history of substance use disorders, comorbid psychiatric illness, exposure to parental and peer use, and poor academic performance.[4–9] The type of substance used by

[a] Department of Psychiatry, Massachusetts General Hospital, 55 Fruit Street, Boston, MA 02114, USA
[b] MassGeneral for Children at North Shore Medical Center, 57 Highland Avenue, Salem, MA 01970, USA
[c] Pediatric Psychopharmacology Clinic, Massachusetts General Hospital, 55 Fruit Street, Boston, MA 02114, USA
[d] Harvard Medical School
* Corresponding author.
E-mail address: ayule@partners.org

Child Adolesc Psychiatric Clin N Am 21 (2012) 175–186
doi:10.1016/j.chc.2011.09.003
1056-4993/12/$ – see front matter © 2012 Elsevier Inc. All rights reserved.
childpsych.theclinics.com

adolescents also progresses in stages and typically begins with substances that are licit for adults—cigarettes and alcohol—before progressing to marijuana and then other illicit substances.[10]

Although adolescent substance use can significantly impact all areas of adolescent development, the authors focus here on the impact of functioning at school. Adolescents who are intoxicated with alcohol and drugs are not able to learn and are at risk for long-term cognitive problems. Specifically, alcohol use in adolescence is associated with a decline in verbal memory.[11] Cannabis use in adolescence is associated with problems with memory, processing speed, attention, and executive function.[12] In addition to adversely impacting learning, adolescent substance use impairs adolescent emotional development and subsequently affects peer relationships.[13] Students at risk of dropping out and high school dropouts have higher rates of cigarette, marijuana, and alcohol use than their peers.[14] Illegal substances are present in most school environments, and the 2009 Youth Risk Behavior Surveillance Survey found that 22.7% of high school students were offered or given or used an illegal substance on school property.[15] This article briefly reviews school-based prevention programs, school drug policies, clinical signs and symptoms of substance impairment, recommendations for referral and engaging adolescents who are using substances, and treatment interventions for adolescent substance use disorders.

SCHOOL-BASED PREVENTION PROGRAMS

Universal school-based prevention programs have become prominent over the past 25 years in an effort to prevent adolescent substance use disorders.[16] School-based programs have focused on educating children on the effects of drug use and the prevalence of adolescent substance use, and increasing their awareness of the social influences that contribute to the initiation of adolescent alcohol and drug use.[16,17] The most prevalent program nationally has been the Drug Abuse Resistance Education (DARE) program, originally developed in 1983 by the Los Angeles Police Department and the Los Angeles Unified School District.[16] The DARE program was primarily targeted to fifth- and sixth-grade students, before they transitioned to middle school, by police officers who underwent extensive training.[16] Although the DARE program remains popular (in 72% of school districts in the United States in 2009), the efficacy of the program came under scrutiny.[18,19] DARE has been shown to make only a short-term impact on students' knowledge about drugs and minimal impact on decreasing tobacco, alcohol, and marijuana use.[16] Longer term follow-up studies at 5 and 10 years also failed to show sustained impacts on adolescent drug use.[20,21]

In 2001 the federal government mandated the use of evidence-based programs for substance abuse prevention in schools with the passage of the No Child Left Behind legislation.[22] The Substance Abuse and Mental Health Services Administration maintains a registry of prevention programs, the National Registry of Effective Programs and Practices, which serves to help school districts evaluate different prevention programs (www.nrepp.samhsa.gov). A recent nationwide study that sampled 1891 middle schools found that 46.9% of schools used evidence-based drug prevention curriculums, with 19% using Life Skills Training (LST) and Project ALERT.[22]

The LST program works to decrease individual risk factors for substance use by addressing students' knowledge and attitudes about substance use, teaching drug refusal skills, and improving personal self-management and social skills. LST is one of a few programs to address personal self-management skills that include problem-solving; skills to cope with anxiety, anger, frustration; and education on personal behavioral change.[23,24] The program emphasizes skill acquisition through active skills coaching and also uses traditional didactics, group discussions, and classroom demonstrations.[23] The program is delivered over 15 sessions during seventh grade with 10 booster sessions in eighth grade and 5 in ninth grade. Short-term follow-up of the effectiveness of the LST program showed decreased cigarette and marijuana use and decreased frequency of students drinking to intoxication.[25] Long-term follow-up of the program in twelfth grade showed decreased prevalence of students who smoked tobacco monthly, decreased problem drinking, and decreased weekly polydrug use (tobacco, alcohol, and marijuana). More robust long-term follow-up results, including decreased weekly marijuana use, were found in the high-fidelity group that received at least 60% of the LST curriculum.[26]

Another popular drug prevention program, Project ALERT, builds student's motivation to not use drugs and provides skills to help them resist drug use.[27] The program is taught through small-group activities, question-and-answer sessions, role-modeling, and skills practice. The original program was delivered to seventh graders over 8 weekly sessions with 3 booster sessions in eighth grade. Follow-up results collected at the end of eighth grade showed the program significantly decreased initiation of cannabis use. The amount of use by students who were experimenting with tobacco and regularly using cannabis also decreased significantly. The original program did not have an effect, however, on alcohol use in eighth graders.[27] Although the program delayed the onset of cannabis use shortly after the intervention, it was not shown to have long-term impacts on drug use by 10th grade.[27,28] The program was subsequently revised to include 14 sessions, which resulted in decreased rates of tobacco and cannabis initiation as well as decreased rates of alcohol misuse at the end of eighth grade.[29] Concerns about the effectiveness of Project ALERT have been raised because two larger scale studies of Project ALERT did not replicate the program's original findings. St Pierre and colleagues[30] found no impact on substance use after the intervention, and Ringwalt and colleagues[31] only found a decrease in past 30-day use of alcohol. It is unclear why the original results from Project ALERT were not replicated. Generally, the field of prevention program research has struggled with how to best disseminate and implement prevention programs on a larger scale under real-world conditions.[32]

Successful universal drug prevention programs have targeted late elementary school students and middle school students in an effort to prevent early initiation of substance use.[33] Programs that are more interactive rather than didactic have been found to be more effective.[34] Key variables of effective programs include the following:

- Changing student's normative beliefs about the prevalence and acceptability of adolescent substance use. Prevalence data on adolescent substance use from community and national surveys is frequently presented in a game format to accurately demonstrate the true prevalence of use.[24, 32] Small-group discussions about the appropriateness of substance use and testimonials from peer leaders expressing antidrug use opinions also help set a standard for group behavior.[24]
- Increasing drug refusal skills through increased awareness of social pressures to use and concrete drug refusal skills. Films or discussions that demonstrate different types of pressure from peers, parents, adults, and the media are used to help students accurately identify high-risk situations that they may want to avoid.[24] Students also need to learn concrete skills for how to manage situations where there is strong pressure to use. Teaching students specific drug refusal messages and how to effectively express the message is critical.[32] Common refusal skills as described by Nichols and colleagues[35] include saying no, giving a reason for not accepting the substance, making an antidrug

comment, changing the topic, or walking away. Discussions and role-playing are effective ways to practice drug refusal skills.[24]

- Providing booster sessions to supplement the primary curriculum has been shown to be more effective at maintaining long-term gains.[17]

Given the disruptive impact of adolescent substance use in schools, implementation of effective drug prevention programs remains critical to the health of students and the school environment.

THE SCHOOL ENVIRONMENT AND SCHOOL DRUG POLICIES

In addition to universal prevention programs, the general environment at school can help decrease adolescent substance use. Individual students who are strongly connected with school have decreased use of tobacco, alcohol, and marijuana. School connectedness has been gauged by assessing children's level of commitment to school, relationships with teachers, relationships with peers, opportunities to participate, and sense of belonging.[36] Research in middle schools also demonstrated that schools where most students were strongly attached were protective. Students who were not strongly attached to their school were still at lower risk for using alcohol in schools with overall strong student connectedness.[37] This research highlights the importance of individual interactions between students and school staff. Students who can be reengaged are at less risk for substance use and subsequently at lower risk for dropping out of school. Connecting with individual students can also collectively decrease the overall student body risk of early onset substance use.

Clear school drug policies also play an important role in decreasing adolescent substance use. In a study of 104 schools in the state of Washington, students were less likely to report tobacco or alcohol use on school grounds when they perceived harsh penalties if caught.[38] Another equally important factor has been students' perception of how well a school's drug policy is enforced. Consistency between school drug prevention programs and school policies is also helpful, and schools in the state of Washington emphasized abstinence from all substances. Schools also made an effort to communicate the school's drug policy to parents through newsletters and parent orientation night with the hope that parents would enforce similar restrictions outside of school.[38] Common consequences associated with policy violations included parental notification, referrals to school counselors, suspension from school, and encouraged participation in student assistance programs. A review by Evans-Whipp and colleagues[39] found that students with alcohol violations were required to participate in a student assistance program 40% of the time, and students with illicit substance use violations were required to participate in a student assistance program 45% of the time.

CLINICAL SIGNS AND SYMPTOMS OF SUBSTANCE IMPAIRMENT

Teachers, school officials, and school practitioners interact with students longitudinally and may be the first to notice signs of impairment due to adolescent substance use. Changes in academic performance, attendance, peer relations, and behavior should raise concern for a substance abuse problem.[40] Clinicians are often asked to help school staff recognize the signs and symptoms of acute substance intoxication. In addition, students are often unaware of the actual long-term impacts of substance use. Acute symptoms and the long-term consequences associated with substance use are summarized in **Table 1**.

Table 1
Clinical signs and symptoms of substance use

Substance	Acute Intoxication	Long-Term Consequences
Alcohol	Increased talkativeness, impaired judgment and coordination, respiratory depression,[41] decreased inhibition, drowsiness, slurred speech, impaired memory[42]	Risk of seizure or death associated with withdrawal, cognitive dysfunction, depression, liver disease, hypertension[42]
Cannabis	Euphoria, increased relaxation, increased appetite, decreased reaction time, impaired coordination, impaired memory, anxiety,[41] impaired judgment, distortion in visual and time perception[43]	Increased irritability, decreased appetite, agitation, insomnia, and diaphoresis associated with withdrawal, decreased motivation,[43] psychosis, frequent respiratory infections[42]
Cocaine	Euphoria, enlarged pupils, increased alertness, insomnia, agitation, increased blood pressure and heart rate *At higher doses:* tremors, confusion, paranoia, seizures, stroke, acute myocardial infarction, arrhythmia, and sudden death[44]	Weight loss, nasal damage,[42] impaired verbal learning, memory, and attention[45]; dysphoria and sedation associated with acute withdrawal[46]
Dissociative Drugs PCP, salvia, DXM	Modified sense of external reality, euphoria, anxiety, hallucinations, tremors[42,46,47] *At higher doses:* agitation, memory loss, loss of motor function, increased heart rate and blood pressure; *PCP:* constricted pupils, decreased pain perception and vertical nystagmus; *DXM:* slurred speech and dizziness[46]	Psychosis[46]
Hallucinogens LSD, psilocybin, mescaline	Altered state of perception, hallucinations, nausea, decreased appetite,[42] pupil dilation, increased heart rate and blood pressure, piloerection, insomnia, anxiety, seizure[46]	Flashbacks, paranoia[46]
Inhalants	Initial high followed by depression, headache, dizziness, orthostatic hypotension,[46] nausea, slurred speech, loss of motor coordination,[42] sudden death due to cardiac arrhythmia[42,46]	Dry facial skin, frequent skin infections, liver failure,[46] permanent memory impairment[42]
Methamphetamines	Euphoria, increased attention, increased energy, increased libido, anxiety, increased blood pressure, insomnia, paranoia, seizure, stroke[48]	Changes in physical appearance due to malnutrition and poor hygiene including severe dental decay and weight loss, skin picking, skin abscesses, memory loss, psychosis, myocardial infarction, cardiomyopathy, stroke[48]

(continued on next page)

Table 1 (continued)		
Substance	Acute Intoxication	Long-Term Consequences
MDMA (ecstasy)	Euphoria, decreased appetite, sweating, pupil dilation, increased heart rate, decreased or increased blood pressure, hyperthermia,[46] empathic feelings, increased tactile sensitivity, insomnia[42]	Permanent cognitive impairment, teeth grinding and jaw clenching,[46] depression[42]
Nicotine Tobacco	Decreased stress and anxiety, improved concentration, improved reaction time,[49] increased heart rate and blood pressure[42]	Irritability, depressed mood, agitation, and anxiety associated with withdrawal[49]; chronic lung disease, cardiovascular disease, cancer, stroke[42]
Opioids Heroin, hydrocodone, hydromorphone, oxycodone	Euphoria, pain relief, sedation, constricted pupils, impaired attention and memory, slowed movements, decreased heart rate, respiratory depression[46]	Anxiety, insomnia, nausea, vomiting, diarrhea, frequent yawning, dilated pupils, rhinorrhea, piloerection, increased heart rate associated with withdrawal[46]
Sedatives Benzodiazepines, barbiturates	Sedation, decreased anxiety and inhibition, slurred speech, dizziness, impaired motor coordination,[46] poor concentration, impaired memory, decreased heart rate and blood pressure, respiratory depression[50]	Risk of seizure or death associated with physiologic withdrawal[50]
Prescription Stimulants Amphetamines, methylphenidate	Euphoria, increased alertness, increased motor movements, increased heart rate and blood pressure, decreased appetite *At increased doses*: paranoia, cardiac arrhythmia, paranoia[51]	Weight loss, psychosis, aggression[50]

Abbreviations: DXM, dextromethorphan; LSD, lysergic acid diethylamide; MDMA, methylenedioxymethamphetamine; PHP, phencyclidine.

DRUG TESTING IN SCHOOLS

Drug testing has become more common in schools since the Supreme Court ruled that it was constitutional to randomly drug test high school student athletes in 1995.[52] Testing was expanded to include middle school and high school students participating in extracurricular activities in 2002.[52] The US Department of Education provides grant funding to support school-based drug testing programs, and a sample of school districts from 2005 found that 14% of school districts were randomly drug-testing students.[53,54] A concerning number of schools, 28%, tested all students instead of restricting testing to students involved in athletics or extracurricular activities.[54]

Schools need to be aware of the limitations of drug testing. Testing is done in clinical settings through urine and blood toxicology, less commonly through hair and saliva testing.[55] Schools commonly use urine drug tests because of convenience and cost. Students who are using substances are highly motivated to adulterate urine samples, and urine tests need to evaluate for dilution and include other measures such as temperature to help insure the validity of the testing.[55] Urine tests vary widely in which drugs can be detected, and school officials and parents need to be aware of the sensitivity of urine samples and the potential for false positives. With the exception of marijuana, most urine tests are at best able to detect substance use within the past 2 to 3 days.[55] Synthetic marijuana and oxycodone, the most commonly used opioid by adolescents, are not detected by most routine urine toxicology screens.[56] The US Department of Education also specifies that schools that perform urine drug testing must have a medical review officer—a licensed physician who is an expert in drug and alcohol testing—review positive tests.[53]

If a school chooses to do drug testing it must be part of a comprehensive drug prevention program, and the school must provide referral to treatment for students identified as drug users while ensuring the confidentiality of testing results.[53] Research by Ringwalt and colleagues[57] indicates that after a student's first positive drug test, the majority of schools notify a school counselor or administrator and the student's parents and provide referrals to substance abuse counseling services. Student drug testing results are supposed to remain confidential in accordance with the Family Educational Rights and Privacy Act and the federal Confidentiality of Alcohol and Drug Abuse Patient Records guidelines.[57] Ringwalt and colleagues'[57] research further found that 45% of schools notified law enforcement officials after a student had a positive drug test, which currently is a violation of student's privacy rights.

WHAT TO DO WHEN CONCERNED THAT A STUDENT IS INTOXICATED OR MAY BE USING SUBSTANCES

Given the complications associated with drug testing and concerns about students' confidentiality, further evaluation of substance use, screening, and continued monitoring may be best done by a child's pediatrician or family practitioner. Schools are well-positioned to help identify students at risk for substance use disorders. Once a substance use problem has been identified, it is helpful for one person at the school to be designated to provide support for the student and to help coordinate with outside providers including a student's pediatrician and psychiatric clinicians.[40] The student's pediatrician and psychiatric clinicians will need to evaluate for comorbid psychiatric illness that could be contributing to the student's substance use, determine the intensity of psychiatric services needed, and continue to monitor for drug use.[40]

When first confronted about substance use, most adolescents do not view themselves as having a problem. Often adolescents view their substance use as normative and have a poor perspective on the true prevalence of substance use among their peers generally. Developmentally, as adolescents become more autonomous they may view substance use as a choice for them to make independent of their parents' or school's rules. Adolescents often want increased independence and freedom, which ironically can be lost when they get into trouble with their parents, school, or the law while using substances.

Lecturing adolescents about the risks associated with their behaviors often increases their resistance to change.[58] A critical component in engaging adolescents to consider changing their behavior involves helping them critically think about their goals and how their substance use impacts their ability to reach their goals. Motivational interviewing (MI) has been shown to be an effective way of interacting with adolescents to engage them in behavioral change. MI is collaborative, elicits the adolescent's inherent motivation for change, and honors autonomy and self-efficacy. MI explores an adolescent's perspective and ambivalence to change with open-ended questions, affirmations, reflective listening, and summaries that emphasize the

Table 2
Examples of motivational interviewing methods

Method	Example
Open-ended questions	• What brought you to the principal's office earlier today? • What do you like about using marijuana? • What do you dislike about using alcohol?
Affirmations	• Thanks for talking with me today. • It was really helpful to hear your perspective.
Reflective listening	• You are angry that I thought you were high. • You are worried about how your parents are going to respond.
Summary statement	• It is important for you to do fun things with your friends. You feel like you only have fun with your friends when you are high. On the other hand, you don't get to see your friends when you are suspended from school or grounded by your parents because of your substance use. What else?

key elements discussed including comments about changing behavior.[58] Examples of MI methods are listed in **Table 2**.

McCambridge and Strang[59] found that single sessions of MI significantly reduced adolescent and young adult use of tobacco, alcohol, and cannabis at 3-month follow-up. MI is a well-suited tool for teachers, counselors, administrators, and school nurses to quickly engage at-risk adolescents in behavioral change. MI can also help school staff maintain a positive relationship with an adolescent while encouraging further evaluation and treatment outside of the school setting.

SUBSTANCE USE TREATMENT

Multiple treatment approaches in various treatment settings exist to treat adolescent substance use disorders. Individual, group, and family interventions have empirical support.[60] Within modalities, no one approach has been shown to be significantly more efficacious then another. Important components for individual treatment according to the American Academy of Child and Adolescent Psychiatry (AACAP) include increasing motivation and engagement in treatment, improving problem-solving and relapse prevention skills, adequate treatment of comorbid psychiatric disorders, and improving prosocial behavior, peer relationships, and academic functioning.[61] The AACAP also emphasizes the importance of family involvement to improve parent and child communication as well as parental supervision and monitoring.[61] Contingency management with an emphasis on positive reinforcement has also been shown to be a helpful adjuvant intervention to improve successful treatment outcomes.[62]

The intensity of treatment is primarily determined by the adolescent's frequency and quantity of substance use, type of substance used, risk of harm to self or others, and willingness to engage in treatment. Treatment can vary from weekly outpatient appointments to intensive outpatient treatment, partial hospitalization, residential hospitalization, inpatient hospitalization, or placement in a longer term therapeutic community. Treatment options are at times limited by program availability and insurance coverage. Adolescents who have inconsistent school attendance or legal involvement because of their substance use and are struggling academically and socially would likely benefit from more intensive treatment such as partial or residential hospitalization. As adolescents engage in treatment, some continue to have conflict with their family, have difficulty changing their substance use behaviors and peer group, or are unable to return to school consistently, and they may need placement in a residential therapeutic community. Alternative treatments to residential programs include outdoor behavioral health care treatment programs (wilderness programs), although there is little research on the efficacy of these programs. When parents unilaterally place their child in these programs, school districts may resist payment, particularly when the programs do not have educational accreditation and are not geographically proximate. Accordingly, families may expand their treatment options by discussing their child's condition with their school district before sending their child to a distant program.

Some adolescents who are struggling with peer pressure and who continue substance use may benefit from a recovery high school. Recovery high schools are designed for students who are recovering from a substance use disorder. Such schools have been increasing in number since the late 1980s. Most recovery schools share building space with another organization or a mainstream school, although efforts are made to minimize contact with nonrecovery high school students.[63] Regular support groups and individual counseling are key components within a recovery high school in addition to the academic curriculum. A recent descriptive study by Moberg and Finch[63] found that students in recovery schools had a significant reduction in substance use.

SUMMARY

Schools play an instrumental role in promoting children's cognitive development as well as their social and emotional development. Substance use interferes with development and impacts not only individual students but the school environment as well. School-wide efforts including the use of evidence-based universal substance use prevention programs, attempts to increase students' attachment to school, and clear school drug policies can decrease early-onset adolescent substance use. It is important for school staff to identify students who are at increased risk for substance use or show signs of substance use and to refer them to their pediatrician or psychiatric clinician for further evaluation. Given the complexities associated with urine drug screening in the school setting, school resources dedicated to decreasing substance use may be better focused on training staff on how to engage students who are using substances with MI and devoting more resources to help staff coordinate with outside providers who are monitoring an adolescent's use and progress in treatment. Many adolescents can successfully decrease their substance use with outpatient treatment. Students who continue to struggle with peer interactions and school attendance may do better with alternative placement in a recovery school or a residential therapeutic community.

REFERENCES

1. Merikangas KR, He JP, Burstein M, et al. Lifetime prevalence of mental disorders in US adolescents: results from the National Comorbidity Survey Replication—Adolescent Supplementation (NCS-A). J Am Acad Child Adolesc Psychiatry 2010;49:980–9.
2. Johnston LD, O'Malley PM, Bachman JG, et al. Monitoring the future national results on adolescent drug use: overview of key findings, 2010. Ann Arbor (MI): Institute for Social Research, The University of Michigan; 2010.
3. Sanchez-Samper X, Knight JR. Drug abuse by adolescents: general considerations. Pediatr Rev 2009;30:83–93.

4. Grant BF, Dawson DA. Age of onset of drug use and its association with DSM-IV drug abuse and dependence: results from the National Longitudinal Alcohol Epidemiologic Survey. J Subst Abuse 1998;10:163–73.

5. Dawson DA, Goldstein RB, Chou SP, et al. Age at first drink and the first incidence of adult-onset DSM-IV alcohol use disorders. Alcohol Clin Exp Res 2008;32:2149–60.

6. Lynskey MT, Agrawal A, Heath AC. Genetically informative research on adolescent substance use: methods, findings, and challenges. J Am Acad Child Adolesc Psychiatry 2010;49:1202–14.

7. Deas D. Adolescent substance abuse and psychiatric comorbidities. J Clin Psychiatry 2006;67(Suppl 7):18–23.

8. Bahr SJ, Hoffmann JP, Yang X. Parental and peer influences on the risk of adolescent drug use J Prim Prev 2005;26:529–51.

9. Hawkins JD, Catalano RE, Miller JY. Risk and protective factors for alcohol and other drug problems in adolescence and early adulthood: implications for substance abuse prevention. Psychol Bull 1992;112:64–105.

10. Kandel DB, Yamaguchi K, Chen K. Stages of progression in drug involvement from adolescence to adulthood: further evidence for the gateway theory. J Stud Alcohol 1992;53:447–57.

11. Hanson KL, Cummins K, Tapert SF, et al. Changes in neuropsychological functioning over 10 years following adolescent substance abuse treatment. Psychol Addict Behav 2011;25:127–42.

12. Jacobus J, Bava S, Cohen-Zion M, et al. Functional consequences of marijuana use in adolescents. Pharmacol Biochem Behav 2009;92:559–65.

13. Wills TA, Walker C, Mendoza D, et al. Behavioral and emotional self-control: relations to substance use in samples of middle and high school students. Psychol Addict Behav 2006;20:265–78.

14. Townsend L, Flisher AJ, King G. A systematic review of the relationship between high school dropout and substance use. Clin Child Fam Psychol Rev 2007;10:295–317.

15. Centers for Disease Control and Prevention. 1991–2009 High School Youth Risk Behavior Survey data. Available at: http://apps.nccd.cdc.gov/youthonline. Accessed July 30, 2011.

16. Ennet ST, Tobler NS, Ringwalt CL, et al. How effective is drug abuse resistance education? A meta-analysis of Project DARE outcome evaluations. Am J Public Health 1994;84:1394–401.

17. Skara S, Sussman S. A review of 25 long-term adolescent tobacco and other drug use prevention program evaluations. Prev Med 2003;37:451–74.

18. Drug Abuse Resistance Education. DARE 2009 annual report. Available at: http://www.dare.org/home/documents/0310DARE_AnnualReport_11WEB_000.pdf. Accessed August 7, 2011.

19. Robert Wood Johnson Foundation. A new D.A.R.E. curriculum gets mixed reviews. Available at: http://www.rwjf.org/pr/product.jsp?id=62828. Published March 17, 2010. Accessed August 1, 2011.

20. Clayton RR, Cattarello AM, Johnstone BM. The effectiveness of Drug Abuse Resistance Education (Project DARE): 5-year follow-up results. Prev Med 1996;25:307–18.

21. Lynam DR, Milich R, Zimmerman R, et al. Project DARE: no effects at 10-year follow-up. J Consult Clin Psychol 1999;67:590–3.

22. Ringwalt C, Vincus AA, Hanley S, et al. The prevalence of evidence-based drug use prevention curricula in U.S. middle schools in 2008. Prev Sci 2011;12:63–9.

23. Botvin GJ, Kantor LW. Preventing alcohol and tobacco use through life skills training: theory, methods, and empirical findings. Alcohol Res Health 2000;24:250–7.

24. Hansen WB. School-based substance abuse prevention: a review of the state of the art in curriculum, 1980–1990. Health Educ Res 1992;7:403–30.

25. Botvin GJ, Baker E, Dusenbury L, et al. Preventing adolescent drug abuse through a multimodal cognitive-behavioral approach: results of a 3-year study. J Consult Clin Psychol 1990;58:437–46.

26. Botvin GJ, Baker E, Dusenbury L, et al. Long-term follow-up results of a randomized drug abuse prevention trial in a white middle-class population. JAMA 1995;273: 1106–12.

27. Ellickson PL, Bell RM. Drug prevention in junior high: a multi-site longitudinal test. Science 1990;2247:1299–305.

28. Ellickson PL, Bell RM, McGuigan K. Preventing adolescent drug use: long-term results of a junior high program. Am J Public Health 1993;83:856–61.

29. Ellickson PL, McCaffrey DF, Ghosh-Dastidar B, et al. New inroads in preventing adolescent drug use: results from a large-scale trial of project ALERT in middle schools. Am J Public Health 2003;93:1830–6.

30. St Pierre TL, Osgood DW, Mincemoyer CC, et al. Results of an independent evaluation of Project ALERT delivered in schools by Cooperative Extension. Prev Sci 2005;6:305–17.

31. Ringwalt CL, Clark HK, Hanley S, et al. Project ALERT: a cluster randomized trial. Arch Pediatr Adolesc Med 2009;163:625–32.

32. Botvin GJ, Griffin KW. School-based programmes to prevent alcohol, tobacco, and other drug use. Int Rev Psychiatry 2007;19:607–15.

33. Gottfredson DC, Wilson DB. Characteristics of effective school-based substance abuse prevention. Prev Sci 2003;4:27–38.

34. Tobler NS, Stratton HH. Effectiveness of school based drug prevention programs: a meta-analysis of the research. J Prim Prevent 1997;18:71–128.

35. Nichols TR, Graber JA, Brooks-Gun J, et al. Ways to say no: refusal skill strategies among urban adolescents. Am J Health Behav 2006;30:227–36.

36. Bond L, Butler H, Thomas L, et al. Social and school connectedness in early secondary school as predictors of late teenage substance use, mental health, and academic outcomes. J Adolesc Health 2007;40:357:e9–e18

37. Henry KL, Slater MD. The contextual effect of school attachment on young adolescents' alcohol use. J Sch Health 2007;77:67–74.

38. Evans-Whipp TJ, Bond L, Toumbourou JW, et al. School, parent, and student perspectives of school drug policies. J Sch Health 2007;77:138–46.

39. Evans-Whipp TJ, Beyers JM, Lloyd S, et al. A review of school drug policies and their impact on youth substance use. Health Promot Int 2004;19:227–34.

40. American Academy of Pediatrics, Council on School Health, Committee on Substance Abuse. The role of schools in combating illicit substance abuse. Pediatrics 2007;120:1379–84.

41. Pitzele HZ, Tolia VM. Twenty per hour: altered mental status due to ethanol abuse and withdrawal. Emerg Med Clin North Am 2010;28:683–705.

42. Commonly abused drugs. National Institutes of Health, National Institute on Drug Abuse. Available at: http://www.drugabuse.gov/DrugPages/DrugsofAbuse.html. Accessed July 30, 2011.

43. Gruber AJ, Pope HG. Marijuana use among adolescents. Pediatr Clin North Am 2002;49:389–413.

44. Cregler LL, Mark H. Medical complications of cocaine abuse. N Eng J Med 1986;315: 1495–500.

45. Kosten TR, Sofuoglu M, Gardner TJ. Clinical management: cocaine. In: Galanter M, Kleber HD, editors. The American Psychiatric Publishing textbook of substance abuse treatment. 4th edition. Washington, DC: American Psychiatric Publishing, Inc; 2008. p. 157–8.

46. Greene JP, Ahrendt D, Stafford EM. Adolescent abuse of other drugs. Adolesc Med Clin 2006;17:283–318.

47. Richardson WH, Slone CM, Michels JC. Herbal drugs of abuse: an emerging problem. Emerg Med Clin North Am 2007;25:435–57.

48. Winslow BT, Voorhees KI, Pehl KA. Methamphetamine abuse. Am Fam Physician 2007;76:1169–74.

49. Benowitz NL. Mechanisms of disease: nicotine addiction. N Engl J Med 2010;362:2295–303.

50. Selected prescription drugs with potential for abuse. National Institute on Drug Abuse, US Department of Health and Human Services, National Institutes of Health. Available at: http://www.nida.nih.gov/PDF/PrescriptionDrugs.pdf. Accessed July 30, 2011.

51. Caplan JP, Epstein LA, Quinn DK, et al. Neuropsychiatric effects of prescription drug abuse. Neuropsychol Rev 2007;17:363–80.

52. Committee on Substance Abuse, American Academy of Pediatrics; Council on School Health, American Academy of Pediatrics, Knight JR, Mears CJ. Testing for drugs of abuse in children and adolescents: addendum—testing in schools and at home. Pediatrics 2007;119:627–30.

53. School-based student drug-testing programs. U.S. Department of Education. Available at: www2.ed.gov/programs/drugtesting/index.html. Accessed August 3, 2011.

54. Ringwalt C, Vincus AA, Ennett ST, et al. Random drug testing in US public school districts. Am J Public Health 2008;98:826–8.

55. Casavant MJ. Urine drug screening in adolescents. Pediatr Clin North Am 2002;49:317–27.

56. Jaffee WB, Trucco E, Teter C, et al. Ensuring validity in urine drug testing. Psychiatr Serv 2008;59:140–2.

57. Ringwalt C, Vincus AA, Ennett ST, et al. Responses to positive results from suspicionless or random drug tests in U.S. public school districts. J Sch Health 2009;79:177–83.

58. Erickson SJ, Gerstle M, Feldstein SW. Brief interventions and motivational interviewing with children, adolescents, and their parents in pediatric health care settings. Arch Pediatr Adolesc Med 2005;159:1173–80.

59. McCambridge J, Strang J. The efficacy of single-session motivational interviewing in reducing drug consumption and perceptions of drug-related risk and harm among young people: results from a multi-site cluster randomized trial. Addiction 2001;99:39–52.

60. Waldron HB, Turner CW. Evidence-based psychosocial treatments for adolescent substance abuse. J Clin Child Adolesc Psychol 2008;37:238–61.

61. Bukstein OG, Bernet W, Arnold V, et al. Practice parameter for the assessment and treatment of children and adolescents with substance use disorders. J Am Acad Child Adolesc Psychiatry 2005;44:609–21.

62. Stanger C, Budney AJ. Contingency management approaches for adolescent substance use disorders. Child Adolesc Psychiatr Clin N Am 2010;19:547–62.

63. Moberg DP, Finch AJ. Recovery high schools: a descriptive study of school programs and students. J Groups Addict Recover 2008;2:128–61.

Schooling Students with Psychotic Disorders

Jonathan R. Stevens, MD, MPH[a],*, Jefferson B. Prince, MD[b,c]

KEYWORDS

- Psychosis • Childhood-onset schizophrenia • Hallucinations
- School interventions

The term **psychosis** is generally used to describe the abnormal behaviors of children and adolescents with grossly impaired reality testing. Narrowly defined, psychosis denotes the presence of either delusions (false implausible beliefs) or hallucinations (false perceptions that may be visual, auditory, or tactile). Broader definitions of psychosis include manifestations of thought disorder, behavioral disorganization, and catatonia.[1,2]

When evaluating a child who is exhibiting psychotic symptoms, a common (and often unspoken) fear among families is that the child is developing or will be diagnosed with schizophrenia. Fortunately, most forms of psychosis in children and adolescents are not due to schizophrenia. Schizophrenia is a chronic psychotic disorder, with an estimated 0.46% prevalence worldwide.[2] The onset of schizophrenia is generally between the ages of 14 and 35 years, with 50% of cases diagnosed before the age of 25 years.[3]

Childhood-onset schizophrenia (COS) is a virulent form of psychotic disorder that occurs at age 12 years or younger and is often chronic and debilitating.[4] The definition of childhood schizophrenia has evolved over time and is now believed to be a childhood version of the same disorder exhibited in adolescents and adults. Compared to adult-onset schizophrenia, COS is rare, occurring in fewer than 1 in 10,000 children; fewer than 1% of patients with schizophrenia are diagnosed in childhood.[4–7]

The term psychosis refers to a group of disorders that impair a person's sense of reality and may lead to changes in his or her mood. In children and adolescents some of the early warning signs of psychosis that may present at school include:

The authors have nothing to disclose

[a] Pediatric Inpatient Psychiatry Unit, MassGeneral for Children at North Shore, Medical Center, 500 Lynnfield Street, Lynn, MA 01904, USA

[b] Child Psychiatry, MassGeneral for Children at North Shore Medical Center, 57 Highland Avenue, Salem, MA, USA

[c] Child Psychiatry, Massachusetts General Hospital, Yawkey 6A, 55 Fruit Street, Boston, MA 02114, USA

* Corresponding author.

E-mail address: jstevens@partners.org

Child Adolesc Psychiatric Clin N Am 21 (2012) 187–200
doi:10.1016/j.chc.2011.09.008
1056-4993/12/$ – see front matter © 2012 Published by Elsevier Inc.

- Changes in thinking: difficulty in concentrating, poor memory, preoccupation with odd ideas, increased suspiciousness
- Changes in mood: lack of emotional response, rapid mood changes, and inappropriate moods
- Changes in behavior: odd or unusual behavior
- Physical changes: sleep disturbance or excessive sleep and loss of energy
- Social changes: withdrawal or isolation from friends and family
- Changes in functioning: decline in school or work performance
- Students' perceptions can be affected by hallucinations (most commonly auditory) and their thinking may seem confused, slowed down, or speeded up.
- Students may have persistent false beliefs known as delusions or they may be suspicious or paranoid. These symptoms vary for each person and may change over time.
- Psychosis may begin in adolescence. It can happen to anyone but, like most other illnesses, it can be treated.

EVALUATING PSYCHOTIC SYMPTOMS IN STUDENTS

Because educating a child with psychosis is particularly difficult in school settings, clarification of potential underlying causes, which may be treatable, warrants consideration and discussion with families. In the school setting it is essential to recognize that psychosis in childhood occurs more often as part of other primary psychiatric conditions (ie, major depression, bipolar disorder, posttraumatic stress disorder [PTSD], or autism) than COS. The manifestation of psychosis in childhood may range from isolated and transient hallucinations (typically auditory) associated with posttraumatic dissociative stress, to grandiose delusions in the manic phase of bipolar disorder, or persecutory delusions stemming from substance intoxication or withdrawal. **Box 1** lists primary psychiatric disorders that may be accompanied by psychosis. Differentiating COS from other disorders is a crucial and often difficult diagnostic task. For example, pediatric patients with bipolar disorder commonly experience hallucinations and delusions, but also have the clinical characteristics of mania, depression, or both.[8]

In children with psychogical trauma–related hallucinations (typically associated with nightmares and trance-like states), psychotic symptoms may quickly abate with psychotherapeutic or social interventions.[9] Compared to traumatized children, children with schizophrenia are more likely to display a formal thought disorder, negative symptomatology, and impulsive aggression.

Because there are many children with autism spectrum disorders (ASDs), it is important to recognize that a number of these children experience psychosis. Like children with COS, those with ASD may also have odd beliefs (eg, believing that they are able to communicate with valued inanimate toys). Children with milder forms of autism (eg, Asperger syndrome) may be misdiagnosed with psychosis as a result of their idiosyncratic beliefs, social awkwardness, and concreteness of thought. Clinical history helps to disentangle these diagnostic dilemmas; the age at onset of ASD (as well as attention-deficit/hyperactivity disorder [ADHD] and speech and language disorders) is usually well before schizophrenia typically emerges. Hallucinations in ASD often occur during periods of increased psychic stress (eg, a child "seeing" a frightening face in the window when it is dark, an experience that does not plague the child during the day when anxiety is muted).

> **Box 1**
> **Pediatric psychiatric conditions associated with psychotic episodes**
>
> ○ Alcohol intoxication/withdrawal
> ○ ADHD—rarely
> ○ ASD
> ○ Bipolar disorder
> ○ Brief reactive psychosis
> ○ Catatonia
> ○ Delirium
> ○ Delusional disorder
> ○ Factitious disorders
> ○ Major depressive disorder (MDD)
> ○ Malingering
> ○ Obsessive–compulsive disorder (OCD)
> ○ Parasomnias
> ○ Personality disorders
> ○ PTSD
> ○ Schizoaffective disorder
> ○ Schizophrenia
> ○ Schizophreniform disorder
> ○ Severe stress

Initial Clinical Presentation and Mental Status Examination

In its early phases, psychotic symptoms at school may not be obvious and may manifest in modest changes in academic performance and relationships. In fact, youth often suffer psychosis for a substantial amount of time without indicating its presence to parents, caregivers, or teachers. However, over time the impact becomes greater and concerned families or caregivers most commonly report hallucinations, impaired overall functioning, or social withdrawal. Hence, all children with major mood disorders or those who display abnormal or bizarre behaviors should be queried for the presence of psychosis. A comprehensive psychiatric assessment should include interviews with the child and family, review of records, obtaining information from other involved adults, a detailed description of the presentation and course of the psychotic symptoms, attention to developmental delays (which may suggest a mental disorder), a family psychiatric history, history of abuse/neglect, and a mental status examination.[10]

Often, before the onset of psychosis, children who go on to develop schizophrenia (or COS or both) show aberrant social and cognitive development. This period of time is often referred to as a "prodromal phase" of symptoms and is characterized by progressively withdrawn affect, eccentric behavior, or increased suspiciousness. Prodromal symptoms initially may be misdiagnosed as a depressive disorder.[6] The cognitive deterioration of students with emerging psychosis may be confusing, particularly at school, and these students may show significant decreases (>10 points) on repeated neuropsychological measures. Sometimes this discrepancy is ascribed to the school setting or instruction, when in fact this is more representative of the evolution of the brain disease. Accordingly, when students show global deterioration across multiple classes (rather than doing well in most, and poorly in a few), and when families also recognize that the student appears cognitively slowed or impaired compared to previous functioning, this may indicate progression of the disease more than inappropriate school interventions.

On mental status examination, children with COS may have speech patterns notable for incoherence, loosening of association, tangentiality, overinclusiveness, blocking, echolalia, or neologisms. Although their affect is generally flat or blunted, it may also be silly, goofy, or labile. Tests of orientation or memory are generally intact (which may help the interviewer to distinguish psychotic from delirium). The thought process is almost uniformly concrete, with pronounced difficulties in abstract thinking. Thought content is notable for hallucinations, typically auditory in nature (as with adults). Delusions are common; ideas of reference are the most frequently encountered. Other forms of thought disorder (e.g., perseveration, lost sense of identity, poverty of content, derailment, circumstantiality, audible thoughts) may be identified in children with COS. Moreover, these children rarely show insight about their symptoms, and consequently their judgment is usually compromised and their impulse control (particularly around self-destructive or aggressive impulses) may be especially poor, and should be taken into account in safety and disposition planning.[10]

Environmental Risks—Cannabis Use

It is clear now that "the grass is not greener," as data from six longitudinal studies in five countries have shown that regular cannabis use predicts an increased risk of a schizophrenia diagnosis or of reporting symptoms of psychosis. Early adolescent cannabis use coupled with a specific genetic vulnerability and the developmental changes may increase the risk for the development of schizophrenia.[11] In addition, "synthetic" marijuana agents have recently been associated with the emergence, and persistence, of psychotic symptoms in patients. Accordingly, careful review of substance use, including previously perceived benign agents, should be discussed with students having new-onset psychosis symptoms.

SCHOOL INTERVENTIONS FOR STUDENTS WITH PSYCHOSIS

Psychosis may impact a student's psychosocial functioning through declining grades; thoughts of dropping out of school; changes in relationships with peers, family members, and teachers; reactivity and conflict due to active symptoms (hallucinations or paranoia or due to confusion caused by cogntive impairments of psychosis); trouble maintaining personal hygeine; and loss of participation in previously engaging and fun activities. Psychosocial treatments may include psychoeducation to student or family about condtion and its treatments, and support to adjust to the cogntive impact of the condition and its treatment (often the medications that are necessary cause sedation). In the school community the goals of psychosocial interventions are to:

- Engage the student, family, and treatment team with the school by developing trust and rapport
- Develop strategies that support and enhance reality testing
- Develop strategies that support academic, psychological, and social adjustment
- Develop a monitoring system to reduce likelihood of relapse and to respond if or when it occurs. Especially in the early pahses of establishing appropriate school supports it is crucial to recognize when the school environment is "too much" for

the student and to arrange a "safe" calm and quiet place within the school environemnt that the student can process his or her experiences.
- Identify barriers to treatment
- Support the student's autonomy, relatedness, and competency.

School interventions often involve optimizing the environment to minimize undue stress to the patient, which increases vulnerability to psychotic episodes, and to match the level of stimulation with the patient's level of arousal. Across conditions contributing to psychosis, school staff efforts to identify precipitants surrounding episodes or deterioration can be useful in determining appropriate home and classroom expectations. Parents and other caregivers can help identify the patient's progression toward psychosis, which may provide specific topics for school staff to "check in" with the patient to monitor the patient's reality testing. In addition, specific strategies for addressing both positive (delusions, hallucinations) and negative (withdrawal, decreased interactions) symptoms may be useful. For positive symptoms, anchoring activities with others, as regular parts of the patient's daily routine, may be useful. When a patient with psychotic symptoms is agitated, distressed, or unsure of what is and is not "real," simplifying the environment, decreasing expectations, and diminishing stimulation are often required. For negative symptoms, regular social interactions with others and structured familiar activities (e.g., eating lunch or listening to music) may diminish isolation and have to be carefully configured and supported by staff because these students may be inclined to withdraw or avoid interactions. Student interventions are provided in **Table 1**, based on underlying conditions contributing to the psychotic symptoms.

Cognitive–behavioral therapy (CBT) to evaluate evidence or to think through explanations surrounding patient perceptions can be helpful to alter dysfunctional behaviors. A consistent framework with similar words/techniques used at home, school, and with friends may allow the patient to employ a regular approach to events across settings, diminishing misperceptions of daily life events and interactions.

Although data on psychosocial treatments in youth psychotic disorders in schools are scant, psychosocial treatment remain a mainstay of the overall treatment plan,[7] and school staff have an essential role in caring for a child with psychosis. Psychosocial treatments for students with psychosis usually involve either multimodal treatment programs or specific psychosocial interventions. The multimodal treatments programs have been established in a variety of countries and usually provide a comprehensive array of services including community outreach/early detection efforts; inpatient and outpatient individual, group, or family therapy; and case management.[12] Unfortunately, to date these programs operate outside of the school community and their impact on school functioning has not been investigated. However, these programs have shown significant benefit including reduction of psychotic symptoms and improved quality of life, social relationshiops, and cognition. These benefits have reduced self-harming behaviors, substance use, and trauma related to untreated psychosis and hospitlaization.

A variety of specific psychosocial interventions have been studied including individual CBT, group programming, and family interventions. Individual treatments including supportive therapies and CBT have been shown to reduce symptoms, and CBT in particular has been helpful in reducing auditory hallucinations. In fact, providing youth suffering psychosis with "cognitively oriented" individual psychotherapy appears to help these youth adjust to their condition, resume usual developemntal tasks, as well as improve symptoms of anxiety and depression.[13] CBT can target specific thoughts and beliefs that intensify symptoms and compromise function at

Table 1
School interventions for psychosis symptoms

Condition	Symptom	Interventions
Schizophrenia	Hallucinations	1. Competing activities to diminish preoccupation with the "voices" (eg, listening to music while doing seatwork to diminish noticing voices) 2. Redirection to another activity or even place in the classroom associated with the hallucinations (hierarchy of places often helpful, with reinforcement for remaining as proximate as possible) 3. Continued efforts to "function" mindful that voices may remain present, but with intermittent breaks (eg, trying to do groups of 10 problems, or read in increments of 3 pages, then brief breaks) 4. "Bossing back" voices or visions by clarifying that cannot respond after 2 minutes, so will ignore and proceed with school tasks
	Delusions	1. Correction (often in steps) away from negative attributions toward others (eg, paranoia dismantled gradually by the student observing that other students close to feared staff/student remain safe, then sitting closer with others, then interactions, etc) 2. Functioning amidst delusion ("How can you still do what you need to do here even though you do fear that student/staff?") 3. Assistants/staff/other students accompany psychotic student when exposure to stimuli for delusions (eg, when going to recess, having another student(s) play a desirable game away from troubling stimuli, such as climbing apparatus that student fears will "catch" or swallow the student)
	Withdrawal	1. Starting with familiar/comfortable peers or activities and then moving to new grouping or task 2. Reinforcing for participating with others or in tasks (eg, "points" for questions or responses during activities) 3. Identifying preferred activities and peers and chaining those with additional activities/peers (eg, adding additional student to a game, or transitioning from effective activity slowly to another with same peers, materials already in place 4. Quiet space to
Bipolar disorder	Mania	1. Channeling flight of ideas to paper, then later reviewing the most feasible ideas 2. Limiting student to giving "best two comments" or writing "three best ideas" 3. Working for brief intervals to manage distractibility, and reinforcing on-task efforts 4. Allowing keyboarding (or dictaphone) capture phrases when thoughts are racing 5. Relying on specific others (staff/students) to quantify mania ("you're really 'up' today, about a 9" [on 10-point scale]), and connecting responses to how manic student is ("since a 9, that means we can do X or Y now to see if that helps you get more in the middle")

	Depression	1. Doing small increments/breaking down tasks to decrease feeling overwhelmed 2. Staff assistance (scribing, helping organize thoughts or connections between thoughts) 3. Allowing other means of work completion (eg, can type/dictate schoolwork, can do picture instead of homework, etc)
PTSD	Dissociation	1. Employing a relaxation routine when feeling escalations 2. Identifying hierarchy of staff and peers to access when occurring
	Flashbacks	1. Bossing back or "containing" by limiting time or depth of response to flashback 2. Controlling flashback by writing briefly about it and "filing away" to discuss later 3. Identified staff/peers to check perceptions against
Substance abuse	Distorted perceptions	1. Protocol to go to nurse to assess safety status medically 2. Working with delusions and gently rerouting the energy toward the distortions
Autism or PDD	Rigid thoughts	1. Hierarchy of staff responses or tasks to alter current preoccupation (eg, "okay, you've now told me two things about your cat, please tell me about your neighbor's dog"; "even though you really want to talk more about the train schedule, let's describe where you'd go if you took the early vs late train")
	Self-preoccupation	1. Reinforce efforts to engage with peers (and may require repeated modeling by staff)

school. Part of this process may include establishing a "safe and private space" for the student to decompress initally as practice with CBT techniques can then more easily be internalized and generalized. Although the exact program should be tailored to the situation and "practice makes permanent," the more specific and frequent the practice sessions are, the more likely they will take hold and be helpful to the student. Group therapy can also be utilized to provide psychoeducation or focus on coping styles, stress reduction, relaxation, and relationships.

Family intervention program have emphasized psychoeducation, identification of warning signs, stress management, the importance of attributing maladaptive behavior to the illness rather than to "bad behaviors"or "laziness," communication skills training, and reduction of high expressed emotion, meaning decreasing criticism, hostility, and overinvolvement. School staff can implement similar appraoches to students with psychosis by educating teachers about the condition and its treatment; by facilitating communication among the student, family, and teachers; and by creating a safe quiet place the student can go if overwhelmed by sensory input, either from school or from internal stimuli not always apparent to school staff.

Vocational rehabilitation involves assessment of work skills and interests, development of these skills, and matching people with appropriate occupational tasks. The focus is to support the student's autonomy, enhance social connectedness, and develop competency.

SCHOOL RESPONSE TO A STUDENT WITH PSYCHOSIS
What to Do as a Team

- Stay connected: Do not allow child or staff fears to break down ties with the student.
- Stay positive: It can be very hard for these children to manage their unruly brains. Provide reassurance that it is possible and that there is help for them.
- Remember that children dealing with psychosis are children first, and often unable to understand their perceptions, or why they are changing so differently from peers.
- Refer children who show early warning signs to mental health clinicians.

Roles of Teachers and Support Staff

- Break tasks down into smaller pieces, minimize distractions, and have a plan to redirect the student to help him or her return to the task at hand.
- Give short, concise directions.
- Assist the student with planning and organizational skills.
- Provide modifications and accommodations to the school program (eg, Individualized Education Program [IEP]) as needed, and recognize these may shift or change, sometimes within months.
- Provide support with social problems (eg, difficulty integrating into the student community, isolation from peers).

Roles of School Administrators

- Provide professional development for staff.
- Collaborate with parents/caregivers and community resources.
- Modify the student's school day based on waxing and waning of symptoms during the school year; if the student becomes actively and profoundly psychotic and paranoid about staff and peers, it may be preferable to decrease

exposures at that moment, or even provide home tutoring (preferably for short intervals [weeks] until the student is more stable and the benefits from being at school exceed the risks of increased alienation or distrust.

PRACTICAL APPLICATION OF TECHNIQUES TO ADDRESS PSYCHOSIS
Psychoeducation

Through providing psychoeducation about psychosis, clinicians and school staff may develop a clearer picture of how the student understands his or her illness, with the aim of building a shared model of his or her difficulties, meaning which factors in the student's life are malleable and open to change, which are not, and how these might influence current or future experience.[14] This understanding may guide educational and CBT interventions:

- Clinicians and school staff may "decatastrophize" the experience of psychosis; although it is a serious medical condition, it does not preclude the student from many "normal" and "usual" developmental activities with peers. The student can learn ways to (re)connect with valued aspects of and people in his or her life.
- Discuss with the family and then student what psychosis is, conditions in which it occurs, and the role of neurobiology and experience so that everyone better understands this student's **disease**. Discuss aspects of the student's life that may increase the risk of psychotic episodes, such as withdrawal; substance abuse; and conflict with family, peers, or school staff. Also identify the student's strengths and resources that may diminish this episode and decrease risks of developing another episode.
- Describe the stress response, with particular attention given to the vulnerability of the student. Describe any factors that the student thinks may have increased vulnerability to developing this episode of psychosis. The objective is for the student to identify patterns or precipitants that contribute to psychotic symptoms.

When discussing potential changes with the student or the family, clinicians or school staff may be ambivalent or experience fears about trying to make any changes. Explore what is important to the student and family by asking open-ended questions, by acknowledging and affirming the efforts the student and the family are already making, listening carefully, and reflecting back what is heard from the student and family as the most important thing **now** (whenever in doubt of what to do, listen) and lastly by providing summaries of staff understanding of the main concerns. As a part of this collaborative exploration, a **change process balance sheet**[15] with the student may be created by listing:

- The negative consequences of experiencing his or her current problem
- The positive consequences of experiencing his or her current problem
- The personal benefits that may come if changes are made
- The personal costs that may be necessary around these changes.

Once these topics are addressed, the student may be better able to rate how important making this change is at this point, and how confident the student feels about making the change. The student can be asked to rate these items using a scale from 1 (least) to 10 (most). Because the student identifies the areas for change, the student is likely to be more invested, even if fearful or lacking confidence to make changes successfully. The process becomes a collaborative dialogue about the ways the school can help support students making changes as well as increasing everyone's confidence and even competence. The efforts to produce meaningful changes become a mutual journey.

Enhancing Existing Coping Strategies

Staff can assist with taking inventory of the student's current coping strategies: "When you hear voices, how do you respond?" Staff can then help identify which coping skills are effective and ineffective. Students with psychosis may use the following types of coping skills[15]:

- **Cognitive strategies**, such as distraction (vs attending), shifting attention by either narrowing or expanding the range of attention. Narrowing the range involves precisely describing a circumscribed area of experience that may include thoughts, feelings, or bodily sensations; expanding the range involves widening the circle of observation. For example, while having hallucinations, the student may practice shifting the focus (or at least some of his or her awareness) from the hallucination to the sensation of breath, or the sensation of some area of the body, noticing what sensations are present. This can happen even when the student feels afraid, because even then, the awareness of the fear is not afraid and will not magnify the fear or anxiety. In a similar manner, students can practice expanding their awareness, meaning that when their symptoms are exacerbated, they may connect with the broad aspects of the world. For instance, while hallucinating, the student may notice that "even though I am hallucinating, the grass is still green, the sky is still blue, the sun is still warm. . ." Reconnecting with the stable aspects of the world may be grounding during a time of exacerbated symptoms.
- **Behavioral adaptations**, such as increasing or decreasing social interactions, or isolating or avoiding triggers. It is important for the student to identify a safe haven in the school, a place or office where he or she can go, with permission, to decompress or reconnect.
- **Modifying sensory input** by altering sensory stimulation, for example, head-phones to listen to music (and eliminate other ambient noise), or use of a computer to visually shift, or having tactile activities (from rubbing fur to motor activities such as building).
- **Physiologic strategies:** Teaching and practicing the relaxation response as a part of the daily school experience can profoundly support students' use of their own inner resources, which are still available even though they experience psychotic symptoms.[16] The student (and teacher) may begin by practicing for 2 to 3 minutes twice a day, once at home and once in school, for instance. It may be helpful to encourage youth with psychosis to initially practice with their eyes gently open, but looking down toward the ground, as closing their eyes may make them feel uncomfortable or fearful. Practice time may be increased by 1 minute a week up to the desired time. The commitment is to practice every day, and the out is that if there is a day that is too busy, then practice for as a short a time as you can, but practice. Another helpful physiologic tactic is progressive muscle relaxation. This technique involves being in a quiet place, without interruptions and progressing through a series of cycles of tensing, then relaxing various groups of muscles, noticing and exploring the bodily sensations in both states. You may learn more about the technique and how to practice it through numerous Web sites. Both of these practices are easy to learn and instructions are free.

- Clinicians and school staff may help students develop a **stress or crisis card.** One side may list contact information of physician(s), clinicians, crisis team, and other supports; the other side may describe various healthy coping strategies, supports/resources available to students, and aspects of their lives that may increase or decrease symptoms or their vulnerability.

Cognitive Strategies for Delusions

The aim of this technique is to maintain rapport while investigating how the student's (delusional) beliefs and thoughts influence his or her emotions and ability to function. This effort is a collaborative exploration of the evidence for and against the delusional beliefs designed to gather information, foster understanding, and generate alternative explanations that are healthy and balanced. The initial work is for the student and staff/clinicians to distinguish thoughts, feelings, and body sensations. This may be accomplished by asking the student to describe a recent stressful, but not the most stressful, situation. Then ask: "When this happened, what were you thinking? How did you feel? How did your body feel?" The student then can practice this exercise with new situations. Helping the student to differentiate between thoughts, feelings, body sensations, and the situation helps break down the overwhelming sensations surrounding delusions. The next step is to explore the thoughts and feelings connection by asking questions such as, "Well in this situation, if you were thinking. . .then how might you have felt?" or "In this situation if you felt this way. . .then how would you have thought about it?" Once the student is actively involved in this investigation then, if clinically appropriate, identifying a minor delusional belief and investigating how this belief affects thinking, feelings, and body sensations can be attempted. Staff can ultimately (after working on the minor delusions so that the student is comfortable with this process) consider asking the student to investigate and question more significant delusional beliefs. This challenge may be accomplished using a simple experimental paradigm in which the clinician may gently verbally challenge the student's belief and then search together for an alternative understanding of a specific belief or situation. It may be helpful to maintain an experimental log of the initial beliefs and the challenges and alternative hypotheses. Such exploration should be collaborative and conducted with a focus on maintaining the rapport, while pushing beyond the student's comfort and looking into the challenging zone but not becoming overwhelming. When this work is done at a methodical pace and with a balanced approach it may enhance the student's reality testing.[17]

Cognitive Strategies for Hallucinations

Hallucinations are often simultaneously frightening and confusing. The cognitive model suggests that patients who experience auditory hallucinations have difficulty distinguishing between internal private events such as thoughts and external public events such as voices.[18] Chadwick and colleagues suggest that people's beliefs about their hallucinations are the most powerful influence in producing distress.[19] Therefore, if students believe that the voices are very powerful, out of their control, and want to harm them, then they are likely to experience a great deal of distress. Chadwick and colleagues suggest that it is important to understand the person's beliefs about his or her hallucinations and to record them using a **thought diary.** In this diary the student (and clinician) record:

- What happened during the experience (ie, "I heard voices tell me to do . . .)
- How did you feel?
- How did you respond?

- What were you thinking?
- What did you notice in your body?

After investigating the thoughts, feelings, body sensations, and responses in detail, the process resembles that that for delusions. Disrupting automatic thoughts by addressing underlying beliefs about the voices can be tested by staff. Like working with delusions, this process should be slow paced and balanced to avoid overwhelming the student and making him or her more psychotic, and with attention to exacerbations of hallucinations in frequency or intensity (which may indicate the need for staff to proceed more slowly, with less intense hallucinations initially).

Behavioral Skills Training for Psychosis

Behavioral skills training may expand students' coping strategies. Five techniques may be helpful for students with psychosis[15]:

1. **Relaxation and stress reduction:** The relaxation response and progressive muscle relaxation techniques were described in a previous section. In addition to these, many other tactics are available for promoting relaxation.
2. **Graded exposure:** Develop a distress scale of 1 (not very stressed) to 100 (the most stressed), and use this scale to assess the level of distress experienced as a result of certain activities or situations that the student currently avoids. Students can then better articulate their fears or distress in a tolerable manner and develop a hierarchy of feared situations (cafeteria is a 95 but eating in Dr X's room is a 56). Once this hierarchy is developed, then the less stressful circumstances can be discussed to break down the student's fears into manageable chunks. It is essential to distinguish avoidance that is due to anxiety and when the exposure is "too much" from the feared situation itself. Regularly checking in with students about where on the distress scale they currently feel can guide the pace and intensity of the exposure.
3. **Activity scheduling:** Develop a chart to record the student's activities over the course of a week and carefully review with him or her. Identifyng the student's baseline level of activity can lead to implementing schedule changes to decrease escalations or several precipitants being close together that intensify stress. It may be helpful to rate various experiences on a graph on which one axis represents pleasant and unpleasant activities and the other axis represents the level of accomplishment the student feels.
4. **Distraction:** Survey the landscape of the student's current distractions and work together to pick the most helpful and healthiest one to utilize.
5. **Problem solving and organizational support:** Usually youth with psychosis experience significant impairments in executive functions due to their illness or its treatment. Helping the student, family, and teachers understand the degree of cognitive impairment is helpful to set realistic (and often adjusted) academic goals. Then plans to achieve this can occur (perhaps using a balance sheet of positives and negatives).

Relapse Prevention Strategies

The essential role of school staff in supporting the student may help decrease the likelihood of relapse by[15]:

- Identifying early warning signs
- Developing a plan on how to respond to these early warning signs
- Ensuring interventions by school staff are familiar, clear, open, and collaborative

- Providing flexibility to respond to the student's evolving needs and require-ments. The student's needs may change within or between days; on some days he or she may experience more worry, on others more fear.
- Regularly reviewing of staff and family understanding of the student and what is most important to the school treatment plan
- Responding to psychotic material. This remains important to understand the student's experience and remain an ally with the student as symptoms wax and wane. Listening by inviting details of the student's description of his or her symptoms without endorsing or challenging them, while still pursuing "the facts" can be useful in revising needs for student planning.

WHEN IS IT APPROPRIATE TO CONSIDER A TRANSITION TO A DIFFERENT SCHOOL?

Despite all the diligence of school staff, sometimes the current school placement is not sufficient to meet the student's mental health needs and some students will require placement in day or residential therapeutic programs. These students usually suffer with marked symptoms of psychosis and are not able to function in a healthy manner in their local school setting. Often these youth and their families receive support from the Department of Mental Health. It is crucial to the health of the child to recognize when the current school environment is inadequate to meet the child's needs. This is usually evidenced by the child's severe disruptive behaviors, over-whelming fears, school refusal, aggressive or threatening behaviors, or a general lack of progress or function. In these situations it is important for the educational team, the student, the family, and any involved outside agencies (Department of Mental Health, Department of Children and Family, Department of Youth Services), and the student's health care clinicians, to collaborate and to consider appropriate outside placement. In this process, all team members may help to identify appropriate programs.

REFERENCES

1. American Psychiatric Association. Diagnostic and statistical manual of mental disor-ders. 4th edition, text revision. Washington, DC: American Psychiatric Press; 2000.
2. Freudenreich O. Psychotic disorders: a practical guide. Philadelphia: Lippincott Williams and Wilkins; 2008.
3. Kane JM. Schizophrenia. N Engl J Med 1996;334:34–41.
4. Eggers C, Bunk D, Krause D. Schizophrenia with onset before the age of eleven: clinical characteristics of onset and course. J Autism Dev Disord 2000;30(1):29–38.
5. Saha S, Chant D, Welham J, et al. A systematic review of the prevalence of schizophrenia. PLoS Med 2005;2(5):e141.
6. Schaeffer JL, Ross RG. Childhood-onset schizophrenia: premorbid and prodromal diagnostic and treatment histories. J Am Acad Child Adolesc Psychiatry 2002;41(5): 538–45.
7. Shaw P, Sporn A, Gogtay N, et al. Childhood-onset schizophrenia: a double-blind, randomized clozapine-olanzapine comparison. Arch Gen Psychiatry 2006;63(7): 721–30.
8. Pavuluri MN, Herbener ES, Sweeney JA. Psychotic symptoms in pediatric bipolar disorder. J Affect Disord 2004;80(1):19–28.
9. Kaufman J, Birmaher B, Clayton S, et al. Case study: trauma-related hallucinations. J Am Acad Child Adolesc Psychiatry 1997;36(11):1602–5.
10. American Academy of Child and Adolescent Psychiatry. Practice parameter for the assessment and treatment of children and adolescents with schizophrenia. J Am Acad Child Adolesc Psychiatry. 2001;40 (7 Suppl):4S–23S.

11. Smit F, Bolier L, Cuijpers P. Cannabis use and the risk of later schizophrenia: a review. Addiction 2004;99(4):425–30.
12. Penn DL, Waldheter EJ, Perkins DO, et al. Psychosocial treatment for first-episode psychosis: a research update. Am J Psychiatry 2005;162 (12):2220–32.
13. Bird V, Premkumar P, Kendall T, et al. Early intervention services, cognitive-behavioural therapy and family intervention in early psychosis: systematic review. Br J Psychiatry 2010;197 (12):350–6.
14. Xia J, Merinder LB, Belgamwar MR. Psychoeducation for schizophrenia. Cochrane Database Syst Rev 2011;(6):CD002831.
15. Smith L, Nathan P, Juniper U, et al. Cognitive behavioral therapy for psychotic symptoms: a therapist's manual. Perth (Australia): Centre for Clinical Interventions; 2003.
16. Benson H. Available at: www.relaxationresponse.org/. Accessed October 19, 2011.
17. Garety P, Freeman D. Cognitive approaches to delusions: a critical review of theories and evidence. Br J Clin Psychol 1999;38(2):113–54.
18. Garety P, Kuipers E, Fowler D, et al. A cognitive model for the positive symptoms of psychosis. Psychol Med 2001;31(2):189–95.
19. Chadwick P, Birchwood M, Trower P. Cognitive therapy for delusions, voices and paranoia. 1996; Chichester (UK): John Wiley & Sons.

Index

Note: Page numbers of article titles are in **boldface** type.

Child Adolesc Psychiatric Clin N Am 21 (2012) 201–215
doi:10.1016/S1056-4993(11)00122-2
1056-4993/12/$ – see front matter © 2012 Elsevier Inc. All rights reserved.

childpsych.theclinics.com

Moving?

Make sure your subscription moves with you!

To notify us of your new address, find your **Clinics Account Number** (located on your mailing label above your name), and contact customer service at:

Email: journalscustomerservice-usa@elsevier.com

800-654-2452 (subscribers in the U.S. & Canada)
314-447-8871 (subscribers outside of the U.S. & Canada)

Fax number: 314-447-8029

Elsevier Health Sciences Division
Subscription Customer Service
3251 Riverport Lane
Maryland Heights, MO 63043

*To ensure uninterrupted delivery of your subscription, please notify us at least 4 weeks in advance of move.

Printed and bound by CPI Group (UK) Ltd, Croydon, CR0 4YY

03/10/2024

01040452-0007